The

Daily Dance

Your Guide to Life
Happily Ever After

Safe Journeys,
Sandi

Sandi Athey

DⅰꓷＤ

Distinctively Diva Press
Los Angeles

I would like to gratefully acknowledge all of the writers I have quoted for their wisdom, comfort and inspiration. An exhaustive search was undertaken to determine whether previously published material included in this book required permission to reprint or be quoted. If there has been an error, I deeply apologize and a correction will be made in subsequent editions.

The legal and moral rights of Sandi Athey to be identified as the author of this work and the creator of the intellectual property concepts contained within, including The Daily Dance has been asserted.

Cover Illustration by Tara Hannon © 2012
Dolphins and feather illustrations by Sandi Athey © 2012
Copyright© 2012 by Sandi Athey

Distinctively Diva Press
703 Pier Avenue, Ste B, #309
Hermosa Beach, CA 90254
www.distinctivelydiva.com

Printed in the United States

10 9 8 7 6 5 4 3 2 1

ISBN-978-0-9799902-3-6

*This book is dedicated to those
who love.*

Table of Contents

Preface

Welcome to The Daily Dance™. This book is written with much love for you and your family. For many years I was the host of the Psychic Healing Radio Show and learned that you were interested in learning how to awaken your own inner psychic and live in harmony with the Universe. I called this inter-play with Mother Earth, The Daily Dance™. May you find a warming of your heart, a few a-ha moments, a giggle, or something you just must share with your closest friend.

Here is why I call it The Daily Dance......

The Universe and everything in it must have a positive and negative charge in order to exist. Accordingly, perfection reveals itself in the union of darkness and light; dancing in unison to the music of creation.

This beautiful and fulfilling choreography begins inside each of us. Through our joy and gratitude; we extend our dance card to everyone and everything around us.

Whether salsa, mambo, waltz, or the twist - it's about what turns YOU on. Choose your style and connect to the higher power within you to glide with ease and grace over the dance floor that is.... the infinite Universe.

May your days be filled with all the blessings the Universe has to offer, and safe journeys,

Sandi Athey

May I have this dance? Signed, The Universe

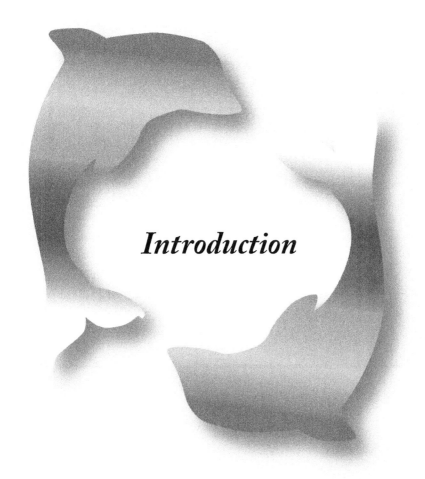

Introduction

The Daily Dance was created with love and is filled with gratitude. So this is where we begin.

Love Makes the World Go Round
Love is the vibe
Where the magic lives

Joy, appreciation, and laughter gives

A heart hope
A body strength
A mind peace
And a life length

Bountiful love to you today from the Daily Dance.

"For prayer is nothing else than being on terms of friendship with God."
Saint Teresa of Avila

Let's Start at the Very Beginning....It's a Very Good Place to Start!

E arth Mother gave me this prayer to use in my work over 10 years ago. I opened every Psychic Healing radio show for over seven years with it. Now, I'd like to use it to open this space. Enjoy!

Father, Creator of the Universe....
Earth Mother, our first and best teacher....
Your children stand here before you in gratitude.
We ask you to guide us to what we need for a positive healing time together.

Teach us that by claiming the health and balance within ourselves, it becomes possible to pass this equilibrium on to our neighbors, friends, family and ultimately our country, our world and the Universe. And so it is for us, our Ancestors, and All Our Relations.
Hey Ho.

Sit back, relax, take a deep breath, and enjoy the magic coming right through this book to YOU right NOW!

About Connecting and Prayer

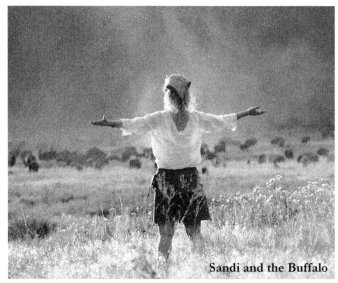

Sandi and the Buffalo

I am confident that with so many beautiful souls connecting to *The Daily Dance*, we will make a positive difference in the energy of the planet, today and forever.

It doesn't matter who you choose to pray with, what religion you choose to be associated with or when you choose to talk with the Creator… what is important is when you do decide to talk with the Creator, get out of the way and let spirit do its job.

When we ask for healing for another, it is best to be neutral as to how that healing is to take place.

When we pray that another person can find strength to change, we need to allow that person's free will concerning how or if they choose to make these changes. When we return thanks for the love and gratitude that is being offered to another and ask that the gift be recognized and used for the highest good, we are lending our support to spirit as it does its job! When we send loving thoughts to another without judgment or criticism, we have allowed that person freedom of choice.

If you are looking for Divine intervention – then get out of the way and let it happen!

"For in the true nature of things, if we rightly consider,
every green tree is far more glorious than if it were made of gold and silver."
Martin Luther

Don't Sit Under the Apple Tree with Anyone Else but Me

P eople often ask me about my "teachers." Well, everything is our teacher.

Everything has a lesson to share and a medicine to offer, when we listen, pay attention and take the medicine as needed.

As I look out my window, I am reminded of one of our most important and beloved teachers ~ the trees. Today we are focusing on the medicine and lessons of the trees.

Trees provide shade, fruit, oxygen, beauty, balance and so much more. They show us how to be rooted in the physical, while reaching for the stars. We all want to be effective, intuitive, strong, connected and balanced. Trees give us this medicine.

If we only reach up for guidance without a grounding wire, our energy becomes erratic and unpredictable. We've all heard about being "grounded." When we charge the battery in our car, we must have both wires connected in order for the energy to flow properly. It's the same with humans.

"One single grateful thought raised to heaven is the most perfect prayer."
G. E. Lessing

Connecting to the Universe

Stand comfortably with the intention to connect to the Positive Universe.

1. Raise your arms, giving your love to the Creation.

2. Call it by name (whatever you feel comfortable with) – Father, Creator, etc.

3. Tell it who you are….this is your son/daughter, _____.
   At this point everything that can be known about you is known by the Creation.

4. Signify your willingness to receive the energy by lowering your hands and saying "Please fill me with what I need."

5. Take a deep breath. Lower your arms and let the energy fill you through your head.

6. Lower you arms toward the Earth, extending your love to her.

7. Call Her by name (whatever you feel comfortable with) – Earth Mother, Mother Nature, etc.

8. Tell Her who you are….this is your son/daughter, _____. At this point everything that can be known about you is known by the Earth Mother.

9. Signify your willingness to receive the energy by raising your hands and saying "Please fill me with what I need."

10. Take a deep breath. Raise your arms and let the energy flow up through your feet.

11. Grab your aura and tuck it into your body.

12. ENJOY THE CONNECTION TO THE POSITIVE UNIVERSE!

Seeing the Big Picture

E agle soared into my awareness today and asked me to share its medicine with you. I'm sure this will resonate with all of us.

Eagle represents a state of grace achieved through hard work, understanding, and a completion of the tests of initiation which result in the taking of one's personal power. It is only through the trial of experiencing the lows in life as well as the highs that we come to see the balance and need for both.

Eagle is reminding us to take heart and gather our courage, for the Universe is presenting us with an opportunity to soar above the mundane levels of our lives. By looking at the overall tapestry, Eagle teaches us to broaden our sense of self beyond the horizon of what is presently visible.

Feed your body, but more importantly feed your soul. Within the realm of Mother Earth and Father Sky, the dance that leads to flight involves the conquering of fear and the willingness to join in the adventure that you are co-creating with the Divine.

If you have been walking in the shadows of former realities, Eagle brings illumination. Eagle teaches you to look higher and to touch Grandfather Sun with your heart, to love the shadow as well as the light. See the beauty in both and you will take flight like the Eagle.

Eagle medicine is the gift we give ourselves to remind us of the freedom of the skies. Eagle asks you to give yourself permission to follow the joy your heart desires.

Fly like an Eagle...let your spirit carry you.

Journal Exercise

I connect to the Universe through:

"Appreciation and humbleness are love notes to the Universe."

Psychic Sandi

The Daily Dance

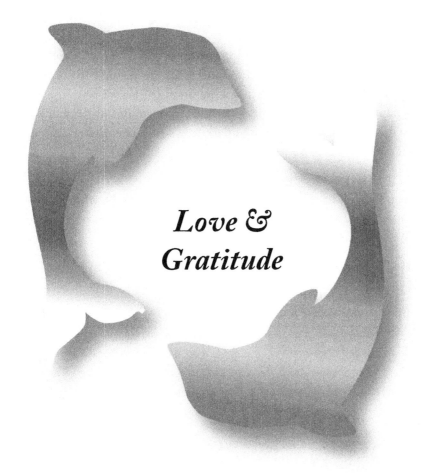

Love &
Gratitude

Universal Balance

Humans are spiritual beings having the physical experience of an earth walk. The physical plane is where we grow, change, and evolve. The Creator gives us this gift so that we may make adjustments to our soul for health and balance. The Universe is all about balance – day and night, light and dark, winter and summer, yin and yang.

Remember, there must be both positive and negative. Don't try to make a judgment as to good or bad – both must be present for balance to occur. Picture the yin yang symbol – when in perfect harmony, the two sides contain elements of the other and they fit together just right. There is darkness in the light and light in the darkness. One side cannot exist without the other for support.

The Yin Yang symbol represents the idealized harmony of energetic forces; equilibrium in the universe. In ancient Taoist texts, white and black represent enlightenment and ignorance, respectively. We may also view these energies as love and fear.

Let's do a balancing exercise right here, right now, to honor Universal balance.

Take a deep breath, clear your mind, and visualize the Universal symbol of balance. The Yin Yang. The two opposing energies or principles, Yin and Yang are depicted in the form of two interlocked tadpole shapes, one white and one black. The white tadpole has a black spot in it and the black tadpole has a white spot in it. The yin-yang symbol expresses the interaction between these two forces; the two spots denote that each principle contains the seed of its opposite, which it will produce through interacting with its opposite.

See them in perfect harmony, creating a never-ending circle of balance. Smooth out any rough edges you may observe, shine it up, and fill it with love. Send it to yourself, your home, your family, your web of friends and acquaintances, and anywhere you would like to experience balance and peace. Now focus on a larger scale…imagining it encompassing the globe and see it expanding into the vastness of the entire Universe, radiating from love inside of you. See the balance. Experience the balance. Be the balance. Have confidence and feel the empowerment that comes from taking action and creating the environment that best serves us all. You must be in balance to dance the love and gratitude step.

14

Let's Talk About Love

L ove makes the world go round. All you need is love. Love heals all. God is love. We've all heard these sayings....but what is love, really?

Love is the highest vibration we can connect to and is associated with the emotions of joy, confidence, acceptance, understanding, forgiveness, abundance, faith, and trust. There is no force more powerful than love. It emanates from Creation and is available to us all. Love melts fear and inspires us to reach our potential by opening our creativity. Being in love does not necessarily mean with another person. It means the heart is open, allowing the constant river of creation to flow through it.

One of the most quoted definitions of love is from the Bible.... "Love is patient, love is kind. It does not envy, it does not boast, it is not proud. Love is not rude, it is not self-seeking, it is not easily angered, it keeps no record of wrongs. Love does not delight in evil but rejoices with the truth. It always protects, always trusts, always hopes, always perseveres." (1 Corinthians 13:5-7).

I'd also like to add that love is easy. Love is confident. Love is gentle. Love is calm. Love is that feeling of peace you get when you are in balance and everything is going your way!

Let's all connect to love and send it out to everyone and everything in the Universe. Through our intention and guided by Creation, that powerful force of love will reach all its desired destinations.

Now, think of certain people, places, or things you would like to join you in this energy and let's send it special delivery. There are a few I would like to mention; all of the animals, my spirit guide, all of my clients, listeners, friends, and family. And especially to you, the reader.

"Gratitude is the memory of the heart."
French Proverb

Where Does Your Love Go?

The Two Wolves

One evening a wise old Cherokee grandfather told his grandson about a battle that was going on inside himself. He said, "My grandson, it is between 2 wolves."

"One is evil: anger, envy, sorrow, regret, greed, arrogance, self-pity, guilt, resentment, inferiority, lies, false pride, superiority and ego..."

"The other is good: joy, peace, love, hope, serenity, humility, kindness, benevolence, empathy, generosity, truth, compassion and faith."

The grandson thought about it for a minute and then asked his grandfather, "Which wolf wins?"

The grandfather simply replied, "The one I feed."

What emotions are you feeding with your love?

Remember, what you feed grows. Feed the positive with your love and attention, and it will grow and flourish!

Journal Exercise

I choose to send my love to:

The Daily Dance

"Gratitude is the most exquisite form of courtesy."
Jacques Maritain

Mind Your Manners

We all respond to manners. The Universe does too! A simple "please" and "thank you" will go a long way. Being genuine with your desires and taking only what you need shows gratitude.

grat•i•tude/grat-i-tood/
Noun: The quality of being thankful; readiness to show appreciation for and to return kindness.

Let's talk about giving praise and gratitude.

I'd like to open with a quote from American Nobel Prize Winning Novelist, William Faulkner, *"Gratitude is a quality similar to electricity: it must be produced, discharged and used up in order to exist at all."* Are you focusing on what you don't have? Complaining about what you want? Concentrating on the aches and pains?

Well, take a breath and look around you. I'll bet there are a number of things staring right back at you that you have neglected to show appreciation for. Every sorrow contains a blessing, every act of life mirrors a lesson and every cloud masks an opportunity.

Look around at all we have been blessed with: this beautiful day filled with sunshine, birds that sing, and life abundant. All of these are gifts. The bountiful earth and all her treasures must be praised and honored for the circle to be complete. When we put out our thanks to our Creator, it sends the signal that we are taking care of what he has already given us. At that point, he is much more apt to spoil us.

And, boy are we spoiled! I would like to put out my appreciation for the air we breath, the food we eat, the water we drink, and special thanks to the plants and animals that give so freely so that we may live.

"Grateful people report higher levels of positive emotions, life satisfaction, vitality, optimism and lower levels of depression and stress. The disposition toward gratitude appears to enhance pleasant feeling states more than it diminishes unpleasant emotions. Grateful people do not deny or ignore the negative aspects of life."
Robert A. Emmons and Michael E. McCullough

Teaching on Gratitude

Robert A. Emmons is a leading researcher in the field of the psychology of gratitude, professor at U.C. Davis and author of four books on the subject. Together with Michael E. McCullough they have conducted a number of experimental studies in the field. Here's a summary of their findings:

1. In an experimental comparison, those who kept gratitude journals on a weekly basis exercised more regularly, reported fewer physical symptoms, felt better about their lives as a whole, and were more optimistic about the upcoming week compared to those who recorded hassles or neutral life events. (Emmons & McCullough, 2003)

2. Participants who kept gratitude lists were more likely to have made progress toward important personal goals (academic, interpersonal and health-based) over a two-month period compared to subjects in the other experimental conditions.

3. A daily self-guided gratitude exercises, with young adults resulted in higher reported levels of positive states of alertness, enthusiasm, determination, attentiveness and energy compared to a focus on hassles or a downward social comparison (ways in which participants thought they were better off than others).

4. Participants in the daily gratitude condition were more likely to report having helped someone with a personal problem or having offered emotional support to another.

5. In a sample of adults with neuro-muscular disease, a 21-day gratitude intervention resulted in greater amounts of high energy positive moods, a greater sense of feeling connected to others, more optimistic ratings of one's life, and better sleep duration and sleep quality, relative to a control group.

6. Children who practice grateful thinking have more positive attitudes toward school and their families. (Fro, Sefick, & Emmons, 2008)

All in all, it looks like practicing gratitude is a good thing!!

Journal Exercises

I am grateful for:

I want to thank the following for the life I have:

*The people who make a difference in your life
are not the ones with the most credentials,
the most money, or the most awards.
They are the ones who care.*

We care, from the Daily Dance.

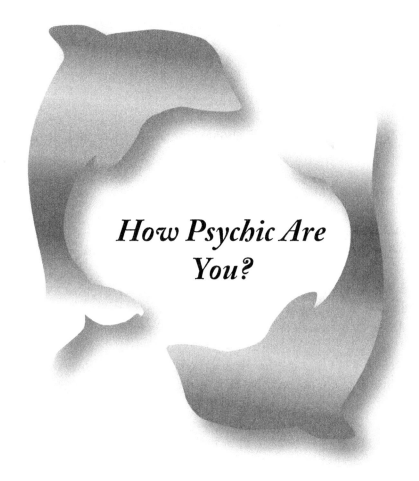

How Psychic Are You?

"Stop acting as if life is a rehearsal. Live this day as if it were your last.
The past is over and gone. The future is not guaranteed."
Wayne Dyer

You Too, Can Do This at Home

Welcome to the how psychic are you chapter of The Daily Dance. This opening was inspired by a very special person in my life...the Judge.

You too, can do this at home.

You often hear people talk about someone or something being very spiritual.

What does it mean to be a "spiritual" person?

Duh...we are ALL spiritual ;) LOL
We are all spiritual beings having a physical earth walk.

Some of the most spiritual people I know don't go to church, don't meditate, don't chant.....don't do a lot of the things we associate with being "spiritual."

Here is what they do that makes them special and shows through how they live their connection to The Creator....

They care
They listen
They act
They honor their word
They say thank you
They create beauty
They understand
They are flexible
They are courageous
They promote others

The Daily Dance

They laugh
They inspire
They compliment
They are honest
They are careful
They live in the moment
They have integrity
They are consistent

It's how we live...every moment, every hour, every day....that counts.

Remember...we are ALL spiritual !

"Life isn't about finding yourself. Life is about creating yourself."
George Bernard Shaw

Picture Perfect

Directions from the Universe for this chapter...

Pay attention to what you're paying attention to.

We sometimes go through our lives automatically. We are creatures of habit and daily routines make us feel comfortable and safe. Take time today to notice what you are focusing on and giving your energy to. Then ask yourself these questions:

- Is it a good addition to the picture of my life that I am creating?
- Does this activity/food/thought/word/action line up with my personal integrity?
- Does this FEEL right to me?
- Is it time to put my attention elsewhere?

When we are deliberate with every precious moment, we can create at will and have all the health, wealth, love, and success we desire.

What will YOU create today?

"Forever is composed of nows."
Emily Dickinson

How Psychic Are You?

Here's the what....

Twenty years ago I was an insurance agent (you can't get any more mainstream than that). Being a professional intuitive was most certainly not on my radar screen. I've learned so much since then and am looking forward to sharing that knowledge with you.

What does being psychic really mean? Is it only about telling the future? Webster's New World Dictionary definition of psychic is simply – "sensitive to forces beyond the physical." Humans have been intrigued by psychic phenomena as far back as recorded history. The first systematic study of ESP was conducted in 1882, when the Society for Psychical Research was founded in London.

By calling it "new age," modern times would have us believe that being psychic, having ESP or intuition is a newly discovered art. Oh....just the contrary!!!! Learning how to control and use your gift of the sixth sense is simply remembering what our souls already know. Just like our other senses of sight, sound, taste, smell, and touch, our "sixth sense" is just that, a sense. We each have it and use it in our own way. The police call it a "hunch," people refer to women's intuition all the time, and you know when your gut reaction to something is spot on. That's being psychic :)

Our ancestors understood and embraced this. And as we remember our connection, hopefully we too will reap the benefits of being in touch with the entirety of ourselves.

Why is it important for me to be psychic?

With cell phones, internet, e-mail, and airplanes...it seems the village of our modern world has become closer. And it has. Because of this close proximity to one another, it's even more important for us to now be deliberate with keeping our own spaces (spiritual, mental, emotional, and physical) as clean and tidy as possible.

Here are a few reasons why being psychic can help YOU!

Heal yourself and others
Change patterns
Bring calmness and serenity

Create blissful relationships
Develop greater communication skills
Attract the man or woman of your dreams

Use your 'gut instinct' to make better decisions
Improve your career choices

Consistently exceed goals
Acquire wealth and abundance

We are all responsible for ourselves and the vibration we send out to the Universe. That's why working with your own intuition and bringing it to its full potential is so important. We all know the expression that the whole is only as strong as its weakest link. Let's all strengthen our links to make a strong and vibrant contribution to our Earth village! So how do you recognize the gift?

Here are a series of questions. Keep track of your answers to see if you have already been in touch with your intuitive self. I'm sure much of this will resonate with you.

- Have you ever walked into a building or house and felt uncomfortable for no apparent reason?
- Have you ever had the feeling that you could or could not trust someone, without really knowing why?
- Have you ever answered the phone knowing who was calling?

- Have you ever verbalized a comment or thought just to have the other person say, "I was just about to say that!"
- Have you ever used your intuition to guide you to your destination rather than using a map?
- Upon waking in the morning, have you ever had an answer to a question that came through your dream state?
- Ever had shivers or goose bumps?
- Do you have hunches that are accurate?
- Have you ever entered a contest knowing you were going to win before the conclusion?
- How about deja vu? Feel like you've been there before?
- Or, have you ever felt that you had met someone before or been in a place before, knowing that you hadn't?

If you answered yes to three or more of these questions, you have experienced and are now recognizing your psychic gift.

Remember to always keep an open mind. At the Edgar Cayce Institute for Intuitive Studies, it was found that the natural tendency for ESP in individuals can be distorted by previous prejudices, thoughts, and conditioning. But when we listen and hear the small voice within our hearts, we can access our greatest potential. So listen, hear, and open yourself up to the possibilities. It is YOUR gift to discover. So, do it in your own way. Keep a journal of these experiences. Write down what you remember of your dreams and discover other ways your personal ability shows itself.

Here are some tips on controlling and using your gift.

First and foremost is how to control and amplify your intuition. The best method for this is meditation. In other words – connection to the Universe. This can be achieved in many, many ways. Find the quiet space inside yourself, cultivate, and nurture it. Practice being in touch with the power greater than yours. It doesn't matter if you call it God, The Creator, The Universe, Buddha, or the force (like in *Star Wars).* Connect to it and make it a part of your day, every day. This could mean setting aside "quiet time," taking a walk, praying, listening to a favorite relaxing song, gardening, or just stopping to take a deep breath.

The way you choose to connect is not as crucial as actually doing it! Establish the connection and practice strengthening your relationship with the Great Mystery. The most important factor in using your gift is that it is to be used for the good of yourself, the Universe, and mankind. Be clear of your intent and reasons as to why you are using these gifts. Remember, what we do and send out can and will return to us. The ancient law of the Great Smoking Mirror still applies; I am another one of yourself. If we do anything harmful to another living thing or human being, we are ultimately doing it to ourselves. The heart's voice leads us to the place of inner peace, where we are in harmony with who and what we are. We know this voice by the serenity it makes us feel and the joy that fills us when we follow the messages it gives. Amazing things can happen when we listen and this intention is pure, honest, and true. *Time Magazine* even devoted an entire issue to Meditation on August 4, 2003 and credited it as a solution to a wide range of illnesses: skin conditions, stress, chronic heart disease, AIDs, and infertility. It even reported that "meditation can sometimes be used to replace Viagra."

It is YOUR gift to discover. So, do it in your own way. Keep a journal of these experiences. Write down what you remember of your dreams and discover other ways your personal ability shows itself. Now that you have discovered how brilliant and talented YOU are.

How do you apply this ancient knowledge and remembering in our world today?

I would like to begin with a quote from Albert Einstein that goes like this – "Out of clutter, find simplicity. From discord, find harmony. In the middle of difficulty lies opportunity."

Our modern world definitely offers us many opportunities to practice what Mr. Einstein was trying to tell us. Amidst the chaos of war, the unnatural toxins in our environment, the diseases, and general dissatisfaction that is running rampant in almost all cultures; we can make a difference and bring peace.

All it takes is for each and every one of us to remember our connection to the Great Spirit. And through that connection, all things are possible. Remembering takes form when human beings come fully alert and aware of all that has come before. The remembering is our psychic abilities, our intuition, our "sixth sense." In order to use the gift with proper intention, you must be connected with the Universe.

The possibilities are as endless as your imagination. John von Neumann, the mathematician and inventor of the computer, once calculated that the human brain can store up to two hundred and eighty quintillion bits of memory. And many call that a conservative figure! Estimates of brain speeds are also exponentially higher than the world's fastest computer!

Oh my gosh! Imagine what we could do, if all of us used our brains! Let's get together to produce harmony and peace for the children and all living things that need to live here. Finding the health and balance in ourselves and then passing it on is the perfect place to start. There is no other time that better suits the self-reckoning, healing process than NOW.

Journal Exercises

I know I'm psychic because:

My gift shows up when:

I choose to use my psychic ability to:

"If you worry about what might be, and wonder what might have been,
you will ignore what is."
Author Unknown

These Are the Good Ol' Days

Lately I've been asked by clients, radio hosts, listeners, and friends to use my gift to tell the future. Can I tell the future? What is the future for them? What is the future for their family? What will happen to the Earth? What will happen if...? What will happen when...? What will happen to who? What is my destiny? We need to know now so we can prepare....

Oh my! Let's all take a breath here, people ;')

The future is NOW everybody.

Our task is not to foresee it, but to enable it.

Slow down and be present in this moment. That is what will create that future you are so focused on. When we keep our attention on this time and space, we strengthen it to move forward in a healthy manner.

Think before you speak.

Listen before you react, contemplate before you think, and most of all....have gratitude and appreciation for what you have before asking for more. This creates a happy now and a prosperous and abundant future for you, your family and all the Universe.

Journal Exercises

What's in YOUR crystal ball for today?

What is great about YOUR Present Life?

True life mastery is more a function of knowing what to want, than knowing how to get what you want.

Form the pictures in your mind....say the words clearly and take action towards your wants and desires.

Leave the how up to the Universe!

Enjoy the abundance! from the Daily Dance

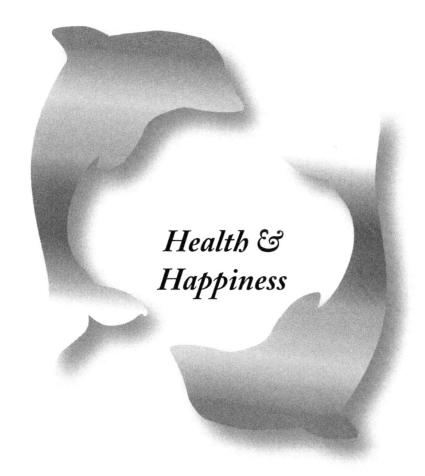

Health &
Happiness

*"Courage is what it takes to stand up and speak; courage is
also what it takes to sit down and listen."*
Winston Churchill

Doin' It Old School

Welcome to the health and happiness chapter. This is where I get VERY traditional and old school. All you need to hold on to is the Universe's healing promise – there is nothing that is done to us or that we do to ourselves that between the Creator and Earth Mother cannot be healed.

Broadcast, believe, and receive it!

Whether it's a health issue, financial issue, or relationship issue, in these uncertain times have faith and go forward with courage, knowing that you have chosen this path and have learned many lessons. Gather up all that confidence and stand strong in who you know you are.

> **cour•age /kur-ij, kuhr-ij] /**
> **Noun: The quality of mind or spirit that enables a person
> to face difficulty, danger, pain, etc., without fear; bravery.**

When you are in doubt, be still, and wait;
when doubt no longer exists for you, then go forward with courage.
So long as mists envelop you, be still;
be still until the sunlight pours through and dispels the mists
-- as it surely will.
Then act with courage.

- Ponca Chief White Eagle (1800's to 1914)

Keep the Arrow on YOU

All healing and change come from within us. Imagine an arrow out in front of you pointing at your power point (for men this is the heart...for women it is slightly lower, near the belly button). Keep that arrow on you at all times so you will always be speaking and acting from that place of power.

The arrow way is the fastest way to know if your attention is focused on you or if it is it focused on someone or something else first. This quick technique will always put you in the driver's seat.

Remember...when you point the finger at someone else...you have three more pointing back at YOU!

Harness your power.

We all have a spiritual space or soul. Some call it our 'aura.' Others refer to it as an 'energy field.' It's really just what makes us special. Like snowflakes, stars, cats or trees, each one is alike, yet each is different. As humans, we all posses qualities that are uniquely 'human.' Yet each of us has a soul that makes us who we are – our personality.

Our lessons and challenges surface through our likes, dislikes, how we have chosen to live, who we associate with and how we view everything. Situations present opportunities for growth. When we take advantage of these opportunities, instead of having to repeat the patterns that don't serve us, we stop illness in its tracks!

Taking responsibility for our thoughts, words and actions, strengthening our connection to the Universe, being aware of our entire being, and having patience with ourselves and others is a great place to start. Often we point fingers at others and assume a 'victim' role. That opens the spiritual space that allows toxins to enter.

Our culture encourages us to be 'victims.' We are told what to do, what to wear, how much to weigh, where to live, who to associate with, and how to take medical care of ourselves. Doctors, clergy, advertisers and politicians are constantly being judgmental with us. When we listen blindly, without questioning them, we have opened ourselves to spiritual toxins.

Eventually these toxins, if left unattended, end up as a physical illness or disease that we can't blame anyone but ourselves for.

Ask questions, do research, pray, find out what works for YOU. And then do it. Use professionals as guides.

The next time you have a problem, sore back, a bad day, or frustration; take a deep breath, relax, be still, and ask yourself how to solve your dilemma.

You may be surprised how much you do know! Like the ancient Chinese proverb says, "prolonged illness can make one a good doctor." The only thing to blindly trust is your own instincts and the Creator. And, of course the stronger THAT connection, the happier and healthier you are. Be patient with yourself and others.

Trust is Everything

The word trust is a noun of Scandinavian origin meaning: assured reliance on the character, ability, strength, or truth of someone or something or one in which confidence is placed.

What better place to put trust than in the Spirit of Creation? We often use the expression "In God we Trust." However, we really don't know HOW to do that. Take your cue from the animals. You can trust a cat to meow and a dog to bark. We know this for sure. The Creator is love, joy, prosperity, abundance, happiness, and light. You can trust that. Hand over whatever you need to be taken care of and it will be done.

Journal Exercise

I choose to connect to:

What Goes Around Comes Around

The Universal Law of Attraction

We have all been using The Universal Law of Attraction at every second and every moment of our lives, but most of us just haven't realized it.

The simplest definition of The Universal Law of Attraction is that "like attracts like." You may also think of yourself as a living magnet. Most importantly, you get what you think about, talk about, and focus on (whether wanted or unwanted).

3 Easy Steps to Manifest all of your Hopes, Dreams, and Desires

BROADCAST - like a radio station to the Universe; our thoughts, words, and actions send a "broadcast" to the Universe. Watch your words and be very mindful of your thoughts and actions. The Universe hears them all. State things in the present tense (I AM, I HAVE, I DO, etc.). Wanting, wishing, and hoping only gets you more wanting, wishing, and hoping. ;') LOL

BELIEVE - The Universe loves us so much that it wants us to be happy and fulfilled. The Creator gave us free will. If we say we have a healthy body - then that's what we get. Know that in your heart of hearts and the rest is easy.

RECEIVE - the best part! Watch for signs that point you in the right direction. Always go where it's EASY and fun - then you know you're headed in the right direction!

Every tomorrow has two handles. We can take hold of it with
the handle of anxiety or the handle of faith.
Henry Ward Beecher

Will Thinking Make It So?

Mind over matter. Bending spoons with your intention. Having that parking space available when you drive up. The love of your life appears, just as you had imagined. Those cancer cells disintegrate and healthy tissue replaces illness without using pills or supplements. Self fulfilling prophecy - what you believe will be. Our state of mental health, what we think, the words we form in our brain all contribute to our well being. After we establish our relationship with the Great Spirit - he/she wants us to be happy, live up to our potential, and have everything our heart desires.

So when we think we'll be happy and healthy forever - we will. Because that is what we're asking for! Taking responsibility for our choices of thought and understanding that we do create what we think about is the first step to mental health.

Send thoughts of love, support, prosperity, and abundance to yourself and others. Picture that business meeting, doctor's appointment, family outing, or creative project the way you wish it to be. And guess what - it will be that way!

Throughout history, the power of the imagination has helped people heal. In Eastern Medicine, envisioning one's well being has always been a large part of the healing process. In Tibetan medicine for example, physicians believe that creating a mental image of the healing god improves one's chances for recovery. The ancient Greeks, including Aristotle and Hippocrates, also had their patients use forms of imagery to help them heal.

Just like anything else, illness does follow a path. It starts in our spiritual selves and if not addressed, progresses to our minds, then emotions, and can end up physical. We have a variety of immune systems and of course everyone knows that an immune system is in place to help us filter toxins, so we stay healthy and happy.

OK, so what are emotional toxins and how do they get in? Being the recipient of emotional blackmail, verbal attack, continued passive-aggressive acts or neglect will negatively affect an individual's emotional immune system. When this system fails....feelings of being overwhelmed, helpless, and hopeless are foremost. It's the illusion that you have no choice that creates the chaos. And chaos is a fertile breeding ground for illness. The seeming lack of choices puts the will or emotional body in denial and that's where we all get in trouble. If locked in that condition, physical illness will most likely be the next step.

Balancing our emotions appropriately while monitoring toxins such as anger, regret, jealously, guilt, shame, and judgment is the first step to healing. Watch yourself when these are present. Do the opposite by replacing them with healing emotions - joy, confidence, acceptance, understanding, forgiveness, fun, faith, and trust. Oh, and of course my favorite - LOVE. God gives us the gift of free will to strengthen our emotional immune system, take advantage of it, use it - it's the best defense.

Free will guarantees non-coercive choice. As Albert Einstein once said, "Everything that is really great and inspiring is created by the individual who can labor in freedom."

We Second that Emotion!

Emotions are powerful, and when used appropriately will change your mood, your day, your situation, your life. Emotions of joy, confidence, happiness, pleasure, anticipation, and love will actually calm you and connect you into the vibration of balance: where all the magic happens.

Sit still right now, in this moment and remember something that has brought you joy and peace.: a child, an animal, a vacation....a smile ;') Hold onto that emotion, carry it through your activities and pass it on to others in your path.

Journal Exercise

I choose to feel:

"I've learned that people will forget what you said, people will forget what you did, but people will never forget how you made them feel."
Maya Angelou

Laughter is the Best Medicine

Human beings love to laugh. The average adult laughs 17 times a day. Humans love to laugh so much that there are actually industries built around laughter. Jokes, sitcoms and comedians are all designed to get us laughing…because laughter feels good. For us it seems so natural, but the funny thing is that humans are one of the only species that laugh. Laughter is actually a complex response that involves many of the same skills used in solving a problem.

Philosopher John Morreall believes that the first human laughter may have begun as a gesture of shared relief at the passing of danger. And since the relaxation that results from a bout of laughter inhibits the biological fight-or-flight response, laughter may indicate trust in one's companions. That's probably why it's the #1 reason women pick men that make them laugh.

Laughter gets rid of fatigue, burns calories, and makes you feel good all over.

"Tell me what you eat, and I will tell you what you are."
Anthelme Brillat-Savarin

Let's Put on the Food Bag

Humans innately desire life. We desire health, energy, well-being, happiness, and wellness. Thus, we should choose that which will bring us the greatest energy, happiness, and health. Since the 5th century BC, people have been telling us a healthy way to live. The way is natural. The way is organic.

When you eat organic foods, you provide your body with vitamins, minerals, love from Earth Mother, and much more. These are the vital foundations for health. Most food sold in stores is grown with pesticides or other toxins. These chemicals have been proven to adversely affect health on all levels. They also pollute the Earth... which affects us all.

Your choices make a huge difference in the quality of your life. What you eat builds and maintains your body and supports the whole....the Earth. When you eat organic you assist to improve the quality of water, soil, air, animals, plants, birds, worms, and other living beings.

Top 7 reasons to eat organic:

1. It tastes better!!!!
2. You are what you eat. (You'll look beautiful!)
3. Food is your best medicine.
4. We prefer life. Organic food is alive!
5. The Earth needs your help. The children need your help.
6. Healthy plants mean healthier soil, water, birds, worms, animals, plants, air, and you.
7. Save Energy.

The natural path honors nature and works in harmony with Mother Earth. As a result, we achieve balanced health and have energy, peace of mind, and wellness. There are many places that are now carrying organic. Big yah! Stay tuned and I'll let you know the ones we like.

Well, here's one now ;') Healthy organic food from the Amazon Rainforest - http://psychicsandi.amazonherb.net/ And remember to say "grace."

The Gift of Our Life

D o we understand and take responsibility for the toxins and chemicals we put on and in our physical bodies? The Creator gives us the physical body and Earth Walk as a gift, along with the Earth Mother to provide for our physical needs. And what do we do? We think we're so smart - we manufacture things for our convenience, thinking they are somehow faster, better, stronger, and more effective than what was given to us: casting aside our gift.

From the moment we are born we're exposed to unnatural substances and situations that tax our immune systems. Powders for diaper rash, bottled milk, and plastic diapers evolve into fast food, prescription drugs, toxic skin care products, and dangerous cleaning agents that are difficult to avoid in our world today.

Our immune systems are breaking down at a rapid pace and what do we do? We create more surgeries, bigger cars, and stronger chemicals in the hope that they will somehow heal us. They only mask the true source of illness. Until we embrace the gifts with gratitude and joy instead of resentment and arrogance we will continue down the same path of sorrow and disease. Our physical bodies do not know how to process mineral oils, but will gladly use aloe vera as a moisturizer and healing agent.

So focus on strengthening your immune system and the next time you have a headache, upset stomach, or physical challenge, embrace the natural pharmacy available to us all. Eat healthy foods, avoid sugars, get plenty of rest, and think twice before reaching for that chemical substitute. Detox your physical body and above all else - be thankful for what you have.

These Are a Few of My Favorite Things

G lowing skin, strong nails, shiny hair, vibrant energy, toned muscles, clear eyes, calm demeanor, quick recovery from injury, low blood pressure, looking years younger....these are just a few of the side effects I've experienced since eating food from the Amazon Rainforest.

Here are some fun facts about the Amazon...and how it relates to you.

More than 20% of Earth's oxygen is produced in this area, thus the name "Lungs of the Planet." We all enjoy breathing.

With 2.5 million square miles, the Amazon rainforest represents 54% of the total rainforests left of the planet.

Amazon rainforest birds account for for at least one third of the world's bird species. More than half of the world's estimated ten million species of plants, animals and insects live in the tropical forest. They all need a home.

70% of plants found to have anti-cancer properties are found only in the rainforest - Earth Mother's pharmacy.

In my experience with the Amazon food, I find that the rainforest literally "calls" certain people. I am like so many others that have been introduced to Amazon Herbs. After trying them, they have become the first things on our shopping list. Check out the site and if they call to you. Call me and we'll do a read to see what would work best for you and your family. The critters love the herbs, too. Gray Kitty's favorite is the illumination blend! The Judge's favorite is the power shake. Una de Gato is my favorite! However, I love them all :')

There are teas, drinks, power shakes, gel caps, skin care, cleaning products, and much more. Ya!!!

Here is the url to my Amazon Herb website - http://psychicsandi. amazonherb.net/ Consume massive herbage!

A Balanced Life

We all have the right to change, to heal and to transform. That's why we have all made the choice to be in the physical world - to grow, change and evolve. I'm encouraging you to DO SOMETHING to help yourself move to health and balance.

Some say "I'm scared." So, let's talk about a specific toxin and one we are all very familiar with: FEAR. Fear is the opposite of love. And everything contains its opposite. When out of balance, fear becomes a destructive and insidious toxin.

Healthy fear comes from a place of non-judgment. Honoring a hurricane by taking shelter shows that you understand what 145 mph winds can do.

The mental human fear is a judgmental, projected anxiety that has no basis in the here and now. Fear is a way to protect our true self from a perceived bad outcome and keeps us from experiencing joy and true connection. All decisions humans make are love or fear based. If we do not make a choice to change, we are choosing to let fate take over and we will no longer control the outcome. Not making a choice is still a choice. Learning the hard way is most definitely the human way and originates from a place of fear.

However, those accidents, illnesses and tragedies create an opportunity for change and healing. When we embrace the challenge with love, we can see all roads ahead of us and make constructive decisions. And love is what propels us forward in a healthy way.

The world was looking for change and was very scared on March 4, 1933 when in Franklin Delono Roosevelt's inaugural speech he reminded us that "there is nothing to fear, but fear itself."

May the Force Be with You

Words are so powerful. When we say we are 'trying' to do something, we are not actually doing it - we are only attempting to do it.

try/trī/
Verb: Make an attempt or effort to do something: "he tried to regain his breath"; "none of them tried very hard"; "he tried the maneuver."
Noun: An effort to accomplish something; an attempt.

Next time you put your attention on accomplishing your dream (whether that is in health, finances, relationships, or life in general), remember what Yoda says, "Do or do not. There is no try."

Have fun doing.

Living in Harmony

We are presented with opportunities every moment we're here to remember how to strengthen and establish our soul's connection to the whole. But, of course, for balance there will always be opposing energetic forces. As we discover alternative actions to combat these toxins, we learn to heal from our higher selves; thus keeping out whatever doesn't serve our growth potential.

Taking responsibility for our thoughts, words, and actions strengthens our connection to the Universe. Being aware of our entire being and having patience with ourselves and others is the key to expansion. Let's all be responsible for our physical body's health by honoring this gift given to us by our Father. Use your body the way he intended and push illness and despair out of your path. Eat real food. Drive by the drive thru. Reach for natural and supportive supplements that actually heal and are in harmony with our Mother, the Earth.

Connect to the Source. Program your mind the way you want things to be. Use your gift of free will and choice often, deliberately, responsibly, and fill that body with healthy, vibrant sources of fuel.

"As your faith is strengthened you will find that there is no longer the need to have a sense of control, that things will flow as they will, and that you will flow with them to your great delight and benefit."
Emmanuel Teney

Another Opportunity for Growth

Challenges in our lives appear as what I like to call Universal pop quizzes. Just when we think we have conquered something, healed something, or mastered something, the Universe puts the exact same issue in our path. Why? Because we need to know for sure that we can handle the situation. And, the only way to know for sure is to take the test.

Instead of getting upset about it, look at it as validation for a job well done. After you take the course the teacher gives a test to see how well you know the material.

I know you'll get an A+.

*"FEAR is an acronym in the English language for False
Evidence Appearing Real."*
Neale Donald Walsh

Pull a Rabbit Out of Your Hat

The rabbit has hopped into this chapter, so I'm sharing its magic with you.

Rabbit is all about fear and how to release it. If you have tried to resolve a situation in your life and are unable to, you may be feeling frozen in motion. This could indicate a time to wait for the forces of the Universe to start moving again. It could also indicate the need to stop and take a rest.

There is always a way out of any situation, because the Universal Force does move on. It is the way in which you handle the problems that allows you to succeed.

Here is the lesson - what you fear the most, you become. Take the "what if" out of your vocabulary and have faith in the future.

"Love is what we were born with. Fear is what we learned here."

Feel the love.

"Be faithful in small things because it is in them that your strength lies."
Mother Teresa

Follow the Yellow Brick Road

D orothy and her travel companions had faith that the wizard would grant their wishes. They held on to that knowing through many obstacles. They followed what they knew for sure.

We are all on the yellow brick road of life. Keep the faith and remember....you always have the power within yourself to make all your dreams come true. Right here....right now. Follow your yellow brick road of what you know for sure and it will be there. Have faith!

faith /fth/
Noun:
1. Confident belief in the truth, value, or trustworthiness of a person, idea, or thing.
2. Belief that does not rest on logical proof or material evidence. See Synonyms at belief, trust.
3. Loyalty to a person or thing; allegiance:

Faith makes all things possible.... love makes all things easy.

Journal Exercises

I have faith in:

I've done a good job on:

*Take a moment right here....right now....to be
in the present. Quiet your mind
and feel love from your heart.
Imagine yourself, your family, your neighborhood,
your city, your country, your planet....in love,
peace and quiet gentleness.*

Be the Change from the Daily Dance

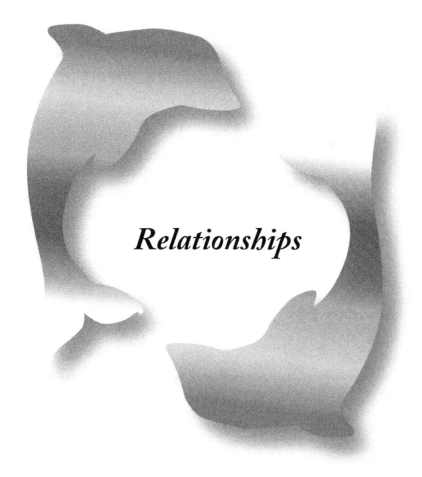

Relationships

This relationship chapter is brought to you by **The Institute for Happily Ever After - Spirit Of The Wind (SOTW), Director**

I thought of you…
When I thought of you…
As I thought of you…
There was love.

Love of a heart healed.
Love of story books.
Love Legends.

~ Sandi Athey

The Daily Dance

"One shoe can change your life."
Cinderella

Let's Talk About Relationships

We are in relationships with everything and everyone in the Universe. How you choose to connect is how the relationship will be. When you have an "eating disorder", your connection to food is out of balance. When you are scared of romance, you are needing to look inside for what is askew in your heart and soul. Remember the law of attraction – how you see and feel about yourself is what you attract.

When you feel healthy and your body is strong, all you want to eat is food that nurtures and supports that. Love is very confident. Love is very gentle. Taking care of your soul, your mind, your emotions, and your body will, by the laws of nature, attract the same back to you. Whether it's food, exercise, friends, or romantic involvement – every connection will be strong and healthy when you are strong and healthy. Like attracts like.

As the FAA says, when the plane gets into trouble and the life saving equipment falls from the upper compartment, you take the oxygen first and then give it to others. Why is that? With only 19 seconds of useful consciousness in such a situation this gives both of you a chance of survival.

We are all connected. By taking care of ourselves in a thoughtful way, we contribute to the whole from a place of balance. When accidents happen, we certainly expect a trained and equipped professional to show up on the scene. This person has taken care of the details, so that we may be helped – he/she taken the oxygen first.

Getting our own needs met is the first step to balance. Knowing our needs and being responsible for fulfilling them is up to each individual. Passing on the balance, which is love, is the goal.

Mother Teresa once said, "If we want a message to be heard, it has got to be sent out. To keep a lamp burning, we have to keep putting oil in it." The oil in the lamp is how we feed ourselves spiritually, mentally, emotionally, and physically. Discover what your needs are spiritually. Connect to the Creator inside of yourself, in whatever way meets your needs. To meet the needs of your brain, think of things that delight you and bring you joy. Remember that thoughts are so persuasive to our well being. What meets your needs emotionally? Align yourself with people, places, and things that evoke feelings of joy, gratitude, trust, and confidence: emotions that build you up and keep you giggling. Physical needs must be present for balance. Meet your body's needs with the most organic and Earth Mother friendly food, water, products, and hugs. Physical touch is so important for us. Enjoy it!

Some think they need to 'do something' or 'have something' to get their needs met and be happy: be that a vacation, a doctor, money, a new car, etc. As Buddha said, "Do not dwell in the past; do not dream of the future, concentrate the mind on the present moment." Concentrate in this moment and think of something that brings you joy. Feel that happiness, relax your body, and enjoy the connection to the Universe. You have successfully taken the oxygen first! Now, pass it on. ;')

"We cannot all do great things. But we can do small
things with great love."
Mother Teresa

And They Lived

Happily ever after is a place inside of YOU. It's a feeling of contentment, peace, calmness, joy and faith.

We often think we need something or someone else to be happy - a new job, a new car, a new love, money, or a new place to live. How many times have you heard someone say "I'll be happy when....."?

Happily ever after is NOW everybody - this moment, this body, this place, this heart.

Live the fairy tale today.

The Daily Dance

"What you see depends mainly on what you look for."
Buddha

Don't I Know You?

Relationships come in many shapes and sizes. We are all in a relationship with every person, place, and thing (as well as with ourselves). When we create and nurture all of our connections, we strengthen the bonds of unity and reap the rewards of peace and contentment. This must begin with us. Only when we find health and balance in ourselves can we pass it on. Almost every person feels a longing for companionship.

From the Edgar Cayce readings concerning the choice of a companion (particularly a life partner):

He believed there were two principles. The first is the principle that we are here on the earth for the purpose of growth and development in consciousness: to grow, change, and evolve. The love impact is most powerful in a marriage relationship and a good union should be founded upon a shared purpose in life and the capacity to help each other grow.

The second principle relates to reincarnation. We, as spiritual beings (or souls), experience our growth in consciousness through a series of lifetimes in physical, human form. In other words, we have been on the earth many times before and more specifically have had close, personal relationships with particular souls. Attraction to another person and thoughts of marriage could very likely be related to memory patterns (even subconscious memories!) of having been with that soul in the distant past. In the readings, Cayce suggests that we are often attracted to a particular person for marriage in this lifetime because of such a spiritual relationship. Two souls may, in a number of reincarnations, grow very close together in their pattern of spiritual evolution. These souls will need the help and assistance of each other as they evolve.

So, did we agree to meet up again with our soul mates to continue growing with them? Are we constantly looking for that yin to our yang? How do we find that special person to complete us? Follow your heart's desire, of course! The Universe will show you the way, if you choose to listen.

"When you find that special person....Remember.....You don't marry someone you can live with, you marry the person you cannot live without."

"The greater our innocence, the greater our strength and the swifter our victory."
Mahatma Gandhi

It's the Little Things

A smile, a hug, a warm thought, a kind word, letting someone go ahead of you in line. These may seem like little things, however when they are done with great love and respect, they become very big things.

We all believe that we must make big grandiose gestures to make a difference. In reality, everything that comes from the space and energy of love makes a difference.

Make a difference today.

Soul-Mates

We have many "Soul-mates" and many people that could be our mate and life long companion. Our souls have met and coupled with many, many others over various lifetimes of relationship adventures. The choice is always up to you.

That one true love is what is called the "split apart". The first ever written reference to each person having a destined mate was given from the ancient Greek philosopher, Plato (427 BC – 348 BC). Plato's theory was that each human being is part of one soul, in which they only have half of. The idea is that the soul was "split apart" and separated from each other and since that time, the two halves have been forever searching for one another in order to join together and regain their sense of original, created wholeness.

Many serious theorists propose that each of these alleged halves of the one soul learns all of life's lessons at their own pace. If the two halves happen to cross paths at some point during life, they may have a powerful bond; because they are each other's "split apart." They find a truly genuine connection. They're so alike in emotions and issues.

I do believe the "split apart" exists. I do believe in true love. History supports this. Recently a couple who was married 72 years and were always together, died holding hands to continue their journey as one. The movie, *The Notebook* brought this to the big screen in a touching and thought provoking way. One of my all-time favorite movies on this subject is *The Butcher's Wife*. I like this movie because it accurately depicts the heart's longing and the knowing that comes when we reunite with our split apart.

Romantics and those in the know have always said "you just know when you know." It's an easy, natural, fulfilling, and gentle connection. Ask Cinderella – "it's right when the shoe fits."

What Does God Look Like?

A kindergarten teacher was observing the children while they drew their art. She would occasionally walk around to see each child's work. As she got to where one little girl was working diligently, the teacher asked what the drawing was. The girl replied, "I'm drawing God." The teacher paused and said, "But honey, no one knows what God looks like." Without missing a beat or looking up from her drawing, the little girl replied, "They will in a minute." Author Unknown

Let your inner child see Spirit today!

Play Date

We put a lot of pressure on ourselves when we are in a relationship. People often refer to it as "work." It takes a lot of work, we're working on our relationship, etc. My advice to you is the opposite – it's fun and it's playful.

The South of the medicine wheel is the place of childlike innocence and humility. It is the home of playfulness and the position of Porcupine. Porcupine has many special qualities, and a very powerful medicine: the power of faith and trust. The power of faith contains within it the ability to move mountains. The power of trust involves trusting that the Great Spirit is always there for you. As children do.

Porcupine is a gentle, loving and non-aggressive creature whose sharp quills are only used when trust is broken. Through understanding the basic nature of this animal, you may come to understand your own need for trust and faith, and for becoming like a child again. Honor the wonder of life and appreciate each day as an adventure of discovery!

Live in the innocence of wonder and joy...using your quills only when necessary. ;')

Now, go out and play!

Relationships and Bubble Baths

About ten years ago I was an editor on a wonderful radio show out of California. The subject of one show was marriage and relationships, and our guest was Larry Hagman of *I Dream of Jeannie* and *Dallas* fame. Larry was celebrating his 50th wedding anniversary and we all wanted to know the secret to longevity and happiness with a significant other. So we asked him. His reply made all of us laugh. However, in the moment, I realized the truth of it. He said the secret was separate bathrooms!

Bathrooms are where you clean yourself, pamper yourself, relieve yourself and take time for yourself before you present your energy to the world. When in a relationship, go to your bathroom and gussy up to present your best to your spouse, your God, your friends, your family, your LIFE!

- Remember to knock on another's bathroom door before you enter. (Respecting the sacred space of another).

- Put the seat down when you're done, guys. ;') (Thinking of other's needs).

- Hang up your towels and wipe out the sink. (Apologize when necessary).

- Girls, organize the feminine paraphernalia! (Some things are better left unsaid).

- Keeping your energy and vibration neat and tidy through what you say and how you feel, invites in healthy relationships.

- In relationships, all the rules of bathroom etiquette apply ;')

Keeping the Arrow on YOU....

Cool Cats

Cats are special creatures, known to be independent, curious, clever, unpredictable, and finicky. Anyone who has a cat or knows a cat can tell you that they have to find just the right food, kitty litter and the perfect environment for their feline friend...or else. ;') LOL

Let's all embrace this medicine. Be finicky with what you put in your body and what you put on your body. Be finicky about your home and your relationships. Know your own needs and meet them whenever possible. This will bring out the inner healer in all of us. This is an important part of the lesson cat shares with us. Cats will only reach out if they are truly in need. Otherwise they heal themselves.

Be discerning and you will purrrrrrr right along.

Meow.

Love Sparkles

Love is a many-faceted jewel that gives humans the strength they need to meet the challenges of life. Every February, across the country, candy, flowers, and gifts are exchanged between loved ones, all in the name of St. Valentine. But who is this mysterious saint and why do we celebrate this holiday? The history of Valentine's Day and its patron saint is shrouded in mystery. But we do know that February has long been a month of romance. St. Valentine's Day, as we know it today, contains vestiges of both Christian and ancient Roman tradition. So, who was Saint Valentine and how did he become associated with this ancient rite?

One legend contends that Valentine was a priest who served during the third century in Rome. When Emperor Claudius ll decided that single men made better soldiers than those with wives and families, he outlawed marriage for young men -- his crop of potential soldiers. Valentine, realizing the injustice of the decree, defied Claudius and continued to perform marriages for young lovers in secret. When Valentine's actions were discovered, Claudius ordered that he be put to death.

According to one legend, Valentine actually sent the first 'valentine' greeting. While in prison, it is believed that Valentine fell in love with a young girl (who may have been his jailor's daughter), who visited him during his confinement. Before his death, it is alleged that he wrote her a letter, which he signed "From your Valentine," an expression that is still in use today.

Although the truth behind the Valentine legends is murky, the stories certainly emphasize his appeal as a sympathetic, heroic, and most importantly, romantic figure. It's no surprise that by the Middle Ages, Valentine was one of the most popular saints in England and France. This story of St. Valentine shows us that if we desire and imagine a loving environment, we invite it to manifest in our lives. Just as he created romance to endure throughout history.

And our romantic quote is from Winnie the Pooh. He said "If there ever comes a day when we can't be together, keep me in your heart, I'll stay there forever."

It's Turtle Time

Today the Universe would like us to pay attention to turtle medicine.

Turtle teaches us how to work with the natural flow of things. Slow and steady wins the race. Too much too soon can upset the balance.

Take your time, be deliberate with your thoughts, words and actions and come out of your shell when the time is right.

Be in step and in time with the Earth.

Find the relationship that works best for you. Be independent and take the oxygen first. Be whole and healthy in yourself. Then let nature take its course.

"Forgiveness is almost a selfish act because of its immense benefits to the one who forgives."
Lawana Blackwell, The Dowry of Miss Lydia Clark

Your Wish Has Been Granted

True life mastery is more a function of knowing what to want, than knowing how to get what you want.

Form the pictures in your mind....say the words clearly and take action towards your wants and desires.

Leave the how up to the Universe!

Enjoy the abundance!

"The weak can never forgive.
Forgiveness is the attribute of the strong."
Mahatma Gandi

Let There Be Light

As I sat on my rock in the river yesterday, I asked The Creator and Earth Mother for a message for all of us; especially concerning the economy.

Dragonfly showed up and sat with me for quite some time, flew away and then came back. So...I looked up its medicine and here it is.

Dragonflies are very ancient with estimates of having been around for over 180 million years! If dragonfly has shown up, you may need some fresh air in regard to something emotional. You may need to gain new perspective or make a change.

When they show up...look for change to occur. Dragonfly works with change in relation to light. Dragonflies remind us that we are light and that light can reflect in powerful ways if we choose to do so. "Let there be light" is the divine prompting to use the creative imagination as a force within your life.

Life is never as it appears, but it is filled with light and color!

When using light, it always reminds me of Nelson Mandela's inaugural speech that quotes a wonderful passage by Marianne Williamson....

"Our deepest fear is not that we are inadequate.
Our deepest fear is that we are powerful beyond measure.
It is our light, not our darkness that most frightens us.
We ask ourselves, Who am I to be brilliant,
gorgeous, talented, fabulous?
Actually, who are you not to be?
You are a child of God.

The Daily Dance

Your playing small does not serve the world.
There is nothing enlightened about shrinking so
that other people won't feel insecure around you.

We are all meant to shine, as children do.
We were born to make manifest the glory
of God that is within us.

It's not just in some of us; it's in everyone.
And as we let our own light shine, we unconsciously
give other people permission to do the same.
As we are liberated from our own fear,
our presence automatically liberates others."

Shine On!

The Daily Dance

*"Imagination is everything. It is the preview of
life's coming attractions."*
Albert Einstein

In the Beginning

Everything physical has its origin in the spirit. The Creator nurtures our soul and when the time is right we become physical. Physical challenges, illness, our desire for loving relationships and the flow of money originates from spirit. So how do we keep our spiritual checkbook in balance, so the desire for financial gain can become reality?

The key is honor, gratitude and trust. To honor the Self is a balancing act that can take much practice. In American Indian Culture, the word sacrifice originally meant "to make sacred." If we honor ourselves, our roles, our abilities and our talents, we must see these things as sacred. When we choose to share those sacred gifts with others, we honor ourselves and those we serve only if we do so without looking for reward, accomplishing each deed with a happy heart.

That's where the following expression comes in – "have a career you love and cherish, do it because you are using your God given talents" and the money will follow.

Having gratitude is the quickest and surest way to add value to your spiritual checkbook. Being thankful for all that is can be challenging as well. Sometimes when we are balancing our physical checkbook we tend to complain about what's going out and we forget to be thankful for what has come in!

Trusting that The Creator, our father and the Earth, our Mother will take care of us is the next step in balancing your spiritual checkbook. If you don't trust them then how can they give you what you need? Just like a scared kitty cat stuck in a tree, if she doesn't trust the fireman will help her get down, then how can he help? Once the trust is established, the kitten walks to the hand and is rescued. Trusting the hand that is stretched out enables the Universe to help us. Trust that the money will be there. Trust the hand of God.

As Martin Luther King, Jr said, "Faith is taking the first step even when you don't see the whole staircase."

Create the financial situation you desire with honor, gratitude, and trust!

"There is no revenge so complete as forgiveness."
Josh Billings

Lights, Camera, Action!

Choices…choices…choices

When we are in public, whether it be at work, on a date or out for dinner…we are on our best behavior. We wear our best clothes to church on Sundays and get our hair done for special occasions.

I'd like to take that one step further to living on camera.

The Creator is always looking through the lens at us.

Let's put on a great show for the Universe!

Let's always look our best, think our best, say our best and act our best. For ourselves, our family, our neighbors, our world and the Universe.

You're on!

"Forgiveness is the key to happiness."
From A Course In Miracles

It's a Beautiful Day In the Neighborhood

S it quietly and feel this prayer of beauty envelope your being and sooth your soul.

As I Walk with Beauty
As I walk, as I walk
The universe is walking with me
In beauty it walks before me
In beauty it walks behind me
In beauty it walks below me
In beauty it walks above me
Beauty is on every side
As I walk, I walk with Beauty.

Traditional Navajo Prayer

Pass it forward.

"When you cease to make a contribution, you begin to die. "
Eleanor Roosevelt

Forgiveness 4 Today

Forgiveness is a healing you do for yourself to improve health and vitality. It is a deep spiritual process that taps on our door of ancient wisdom and remembering.

Remember...the bigger the pain...the bigger the forgiving...the bigger the benefits to YOU!

Forgive someone today and be well.

We all have the tools inside of us for healing ourselves. Our connection to the Creator and The Earth provide us with all we need. I would like you to tap into this space and do a healing on ourselves through forgiveness...

Forgiveness is an attitude that sets us free, so that we are not continually re-victimized by our wounds. Forgiveness replaces fear and isolation with love and connection. Forgiveness is a way to walk in beauty and in balance - without judgment or expectation toward self or others.

Sit back, relax and clear your mind.

Think of one wound that has left you with feelings of hopelessness, helplessness, regret, guilt or anger. It could be a thing, person, incident, or thought pattern inside of you. Focus on that one thing and all the feelings associated with it. Take a deep breath, let it out slowly and let it go out of your body, your emotions, your mind, and your spirit. Do this breathing seven times. Collect all the feelings on the in breath and let them go on the out breath.

Forgiving yourself and others in the way you need to, to heal whatever it is that is bothering you. Feel yourself settle into a new pattern of thought and feeling. Now replace those old moldy, stinky, out of date feelings with the positive reinforcing emotions of joy, happiness, contentment, trust in the higher being, gratitude for the lesson learned and acceptance without judgment. Imagine this new way sweeping in like cleaning day - all sparkly and fresh. Filling all those anxious spaces with calmness and acceptance. Do this by taking seven more breaths. Deep breath in and slowly let it out.

Forgiveness is a healing for you. Any time you need to feel better.

Forgive, forgive, forgive, forgive....

Forgiveness is the subject of many quotations throughout history....I've picked a few to share

Norman Cousins said "Life is an adventure in forgiveness."

And William Shakespeare wrote "pray you now, forget and forgive."

Journal Exercises

I forgive myself for:

I forgive _____ for _____.

Extreme Makeover

"For attractive lips: speak words of kindness.
For lovely eyes: seek out the good in people.
For a slim figure: share your food with the hungry.
For beautiful hair: let the wind style it once in a awhile.
For poise: walk with the knowledge you'll never walk alone."

Thanks to Miss Audrey Hepburn for these great make-over tips!

I have one for you....

For beautiful hands: reach out and touch someone you love.

Walk in Beauty today and always.

The Daily Dance

"The pessimist complains about the wind;
The optimist expects it to change;
And the realist adjusts the sails."
William Arthur Ward

On Going with the Flow

I was guided to remind everyone about the most amazing power that we all have inside of ourselves and that is the power of choice.

Fate is the life path that is predetermined by our lack of attention to our choices.

When we "leave it up to fate" we are giving away our power, thus leaving us extremely vulnerable and forcing us to accept the experiences others dictate for us. When we make conscientious choices, we create destiny and are taking responsibility for our thoughts, words, and actions. In doing so, we knock boredom and stagnation to its knees and weave the web of creativity and growth.

Accessing our potential is truly what being human is all about. I encourage you to take that first step toward balance by making choices that propel you towards health, happiness, joy, and prosperity.

Fate or destiny - which do you choose? Whatever choices you do make, remember to always be connected to the Great Spirit.

As Plato once said "We are twice armed if we fight with faith."

"Horse brings with it new journeys. It will teach you how to ride into new directions to awaken and discover your own freedom and power."
Ted Andrews, Animal Speak: The Spiritual & Magical Powers
of Creatures Great & Small What it Offers

Ride like the Wind

The Universe asked me to share the amazing medicine of the horse with you today.

Humanity made a great leap forward when horse was domesticated, a discovery akin to that of fire. Before horse, humans were earthbound, heavy-laden, and slow creatures indeed. Once humans climbed on horse's back, they were as free and fleet as the wind.

Today we measure the capacity of engines with the term "horsepower"; a reminder of the days when Horse was an honored and highly prized partner with humanity.

"When you feel like you need to move, get out, and break free of restriction, the horse is your ultimate spirit guide. If you've been stuck in a limiting mental sphere or emotionally constrained situation, consult the free-spirited horse." Stefanie Weiss, **Spirit Animals: Unlocking the Secrets of Our Animal Companions**

When the horse enters your life, think about the issues of freedom and travel and exploration. Also, think about boundaries at work or in relationships.

(1) Is it time to assert yourself in some way? Move into a new level of empowerment?

(2) Is it time to move on? Do you need to allow someone else to move on?

(3) Is there any sense of constriction in your life? A need for freedom?

The Daily Dance

"No trauma can be so harsh as that of self-denial and self-repression. It restricts breathing and causes one's heart to ache and one's soul to wither. First, find compassion for yourself and then, extend it to others, especially those who trigger you, those whom you reactively judge in a false attempt to protect yourself. When you extend this heartfelt compassion to others, it will come back to you tenfold. Let that be the source of your freedom and your power. "
Steven D. Farmer, Ph.D, Power Animals:
How to Connect with Your Animal Spirit Guide

Win your Triple Crown!

"I've always thought that people need to feel good about themselves, and I see my roles as offering support to them, to provide some light along the way."
Diana, Princess of Wales

Our Vow to Change

Making resolutions has become as much a tradition during the holidays as getting together with friends and family. Why do we make these vows to change?

Well....What better time to clean out the closets then when the calendar changes to a brand new year? Starting fresh is a grand idea. However, it's very important to remember to take an overview and look at both sides. The month of January is named after Janus. Janus, the Roman god of gates and doors, beginnings and endings was represented with a double-faced head (each looking in opposite directions.) He was worshipped at the beginning of the harvest time, planting, marriage, birth and other types of beginnings, especially the beginnings of important events in a person's life. Janus also represents the transition between primitive life and civilization, between the countryside and the city, peace and war. Reminding us again of the importance of balance. Use Janus's lesson to create a positive connection between last year and this year! Taking into account all that is Creation.

When making any type of change, it's important to remember the fundamental lesson of looking both ways before crossing. Just like crossing the street or turning the car to go in another direction, there are certain things we learned to do before we actually changed our course of action. As children, we stopped, looked, and listened before crossing the street. We often clutched an adult's hand or an older sibling's arm. Driving an automobile is an evolution of mistakes and teachings. That's why teenagers have such high insurance rates. :')

We learn as we go along. We gradually honed the skill of discernment and were allowed to walk to school or to our friend's house by ourselves. As we grow, change and evolve through our Earth Walk, we must honor these teachings. With those new life resolutions, get to know yourself, your limitations, your strengths and your weaknesses, before you attempt to execute that turn. What works for one, may or may not work for another.

It's a Beautiful Morning!

Today is a new day
filled with hopes and dreams.
Promising fulfillment
of all your plans and schemes.

YOU create the reality
of what the future holds
by allowing the Universe
and letting it unfold.

Relax, enjoy, show appreciation
and then;

Watch, look and listen
for clues and right direction.

Take the easy road
where it feels good and safe.
Follow the emotions
that assist you to create.

Make the best of it!

The Daily Dance

"There is nothing to make you like other human beings
so much as doing things for them."
Zora Neale Hurston

Who Cares?

The following is the philosophy of Charles Schultz, creator of the *Peanuts* comic strip.

Name the five wealthiest people in the world.

Name the last five Heisman trophy winners.

Name the last half dozen Academy Award winners
for best actor and actress.

Name the last decade's worth of World Series winners.

How did you do?

The point is, none of us remember the headliners of yesterday. These are no second-rate achievers. They are the best in their fields. But the applause dies. Awards tarnish. Achievements are forgotten. Accolades and certificates are buried with their owners.

Here's another quiz. See how you do on this one:

List a few teachers who aided in your journey through
school.

Name three friends who have helped you through a
difficult time.

Think of a few people who have made you feel
appreciated and special.

Think of five people you enjoy spending time with.

Easier?

The lesson: The people who make a difference in your life are not the ones with the most credentials, the most money, or the most awards. They are the ones who care. We care.

Fore!

I had the honor of being on syndicated radio in Canada. Below is a great excerpt from an e-mail I received from a listener. Perfect analogy for taking responsibility for our life path. Here is the note:

Your radio appearance put it all together for me. It was there, but now I fully understand the path to true awareness and happiness. Everything starts with me. Sandi, what you've discovered is very true in golf.

To become a great golfer, one must learn to accept every shot. I was once playing with a pal of mine who was complaining that he could not buy a break, because so many of his shots ended up positioned poorly. He started saying that God wasn't on his side, and jive like that. Then he hit a shot about two feet from the pin, and wanted me to acknowledge by accepting his high five request. "Man, what a shot..." he said.

When we finished, I told him this:

"Al, until you learn to accept each shot as being your responsibility, you will never learn this game...."

So in golf, you must learn to accept every shot as being yours, not someone else's. And then you become a great golfer.

Thanks, Greg. We appreciate the tips for our game of life!

Hit 'em straight!

"What do we live for if not to make life less difficult for each other?"
George Eliot

Road Trip

We are very goal oriented folks here on Earth.

I'll be happy when I have money, when I have a relationship, when I lose weight, when I have a new job, etc.

The Earth Walk is one long, fun road trip! Most of the fun is the ride. Where you stop on the way...who you talk with on the way...the beautiful scenery out the car window ;')

As you work toward your goals...please remember to enjoy every moment on the scenic highways of life. And take plenty of potty stops ;')

Safe journeys.

Journal Exercises

I'm grateful for these life lessons:

I take responsibility for:

"In the beginning of all things, wisdom and knowledge were with animals; for Tuawa, the One Above, did not speak directly to man. He sent animals to tell man that he showed himself through the beasts, and from them, and from the stars and the sun and moon, man should learn…for all things speak of Tuawa."

Chief Letakos-Lesa of the Pawnees Tribe to Natalie Curtis, circa 1904

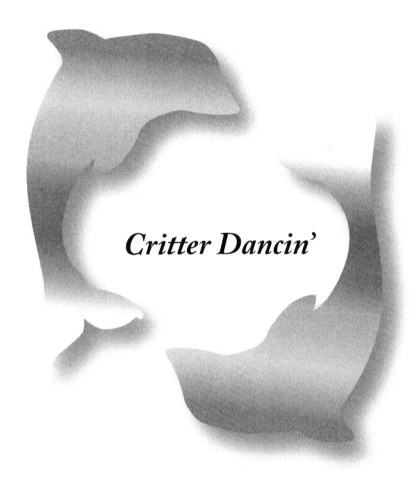

Critter Dancin'

"Success has nothing to do with what you claim in life or accomplish for yourself. It's what you do for others."
Danny Thomas

Sacred Instructions

Native American Commandments

Treat the Earth and all that dwell thereon with respect.
Remain close to the Great Spirit.
Show great respect for your fellow beings.
Work together for the benefit of all Mankind.
Give assistance and kindness wherever needed.
Do what you know to be right.
Look after the well being of mind and body.
Dedicate a share of your efforts to the greater good.
Be truthful and honest at all times.
Take full responsibility for your actions.

Peace be with you.

Hey, He Ain't Heavy, He's My Brother

Hey, he ain't heavy, he's my brother. What does it mean to call someone or something, "brother"? Most of us can agree that by calling anything in our minds and souls "family" we are offering a particular type of energy to the relationship we have chosen to be in. Family means different things to different people. The truth is, we are all family. Humans, animals, plants, the earth, the sun, the sky - everything is connected to everything else. Animals are companions, teachers, friends, and family. Dogs teach us loyalty. Cats bring mystery and magic. Dolphins remind us that healing and community are things that can easily accompany fun and laughter. Our brother, the wolf, shows us how to pick our battles.

- Busy as a bee
- Dog day afternoon
- Sly as a fox
- Eagle eye
- Free as a bird
- Bear hug
- He swims like a fish

We've heard all of these and I'm sure you could think of many more. Isn't it interesting that we eat turkey at Thanksgiving? Turkey's wisdom includes: sacrifice of self for a higher purpose, understanding the gift of giveaway, honoring the Earth Mother and harvest bounties. Instinctively, we take the medicine. Native Americans use the term "medicine" to refer to the special powers the Spirit gives each part of creation: plants, minerals, rocks, and the creatures of the animal kingdom. This medicine increases our connection to the Spirit and can bring us healing, strength, and wisdom. Animals are among the most giving of God's creations. The Native Americans believe that the Great Spirit often sends messages of awareness, guidance, and adjustment through the appearance and actions of Creature Beings in our lives. If you ignore the messages, you fail to utilize a powerful spiritual tool.

When you learn to pay attention to the Creature Beings that cross your path, you will receive much. What were you thinking of when the crow cawed outside the window? What action were you planning when the ant bit your foot? The message will be associated with what is close at hand in your mind and in your life. Learn to recognize your animal helpers and their way of communicating with you. Dogs, in particular, are incredibly generous in their willingness to take on physical illness and even death, for their human friends. When a "pet" passes, it always takes human imbalance with it. The cause of death will tell you the medicine: if heart-related, the human may have been spared a heart attack; if cancer, bitterness and resentment most likely absorbed; if violent, suppressed anger was probably released or a destructive act averted.

When the world was new, the Great Mystery created the Universe to work in harmony. Warriors ceremoniously prepared for the hunt in concert with the balance, asking permission to slay the intended kill. The animal knew of its fate and graciously relented. Every piece of the animal was efficiently used and appreciated. The greed, ego, and possessiveness of human nature has distracted us from remembering our manners - learning to ask permission and saying thank you for a kindness are fundamental and universal rules of etiquette.

On behalf of humans everywhere, I would like to say thank you to the animal world for all you do for us. Thank you for being part of our family.

How to Communicate More Effectively with Our Animal Kin

The reality of spirit beings and their assistance to humans in the physical world is a major part of every religion and belief system. The Greeks communicated to spirits and Gods through oracles. Today we call them priests, shamans, mediums, or medicine people. The Bushmen of Africa developed ritual and ceremony from the movements and activities of animals. Native Americans imitated animals in dance and ritual to strengthen links with spirit. Belief in the spiritual realm is universal. The most common belief is that spiritual guides often use animals to convey their purpose to humans. Animals (and their appearance as spirit guides) can help us recognize our own innate abilities. Their medicines can also be used to help us heal, inspire, and grow.

So, how do we communicate more effectively with our animal kin? In order to have a positive connection with animals, the creation of a relationship without ego is necessary. The relationship must also include silence, respect, and sharing. The silence enables us to truly listen without preconceived ideas. Respect for the lives of others is also necessary. Taking only what is truly needed at the time must be foremost in our thoughts and actions. Sharing is important in any relationship.

Anyone can effectively be "Dr. Doolittle" and talk with the animals. Children often communicate with animals and might even tell you that the dog has a stomach ache or that the kitty likes a particular window. Adults often react to this by saying, "It's just your imagination, dear." You hear this enough as a child and you start to believe that it is "just your imagination." But what is imagination? A big part of "imagination" is imaging, which is exactly what you do to communicate with animals. Animals communicate in pictures, feelings, emotions, and concepts. Sometimes you get a picture of what the animal is trying to communicate, but many times it is an emotion or concept that you pick up. When you are communicating with an animal, picture in your mind what it is you are trying to get them to do or what you are trying to tell them. Send them your emotions and feelings too. Don't worry if your animal friend is getting the right message. If you intend that your message gets there, it will. Use your intention and imagination to get your messages across.

Many times when people are trying to teach a new behavior to an animal, they have a picture in their mind of what it is they don't want the animal to do. For example, you don't want your dog to chase the cat. When you see him eye your cat, you automatically think, "Oh, no, he's going to chase the cat," and a picture comes up of him doing that in your mind. Your dog picks up on your thoughts and pictures and of course, chases the cat. The dog becomes confused when you yell at him for chasing the cat, because he thought he was doing what you wanted.

Instead, picture in your mind a harmonious relationship between your dog and cat. Send your dog pictures of him protecting your cat and maybe even being friends and playing together. If you have trouble using your imagination to create pictures, use words, like "gentle." Just saying "gentle" brings on the feelings and emotions you want to convey to your dog and he will pick that up. Another key is not to try too hard. Sit back, relax, and let the animal's thoughts and feelings come to you. Like any ability, communication needs to be practiced.

If those techniques don't work for you, try tapping into your primal animal body language. Most animals (including humans) use body language to talk with one another. Chimpanzees greet each other by touching hands. Oh my gosh, so do we! :") White-tailed deer show alarm by flicking up their tails. We also stand up and take notice when we are alerted. Dogs stretch their front paws out in front of them and lower their bodies when they want to play. We too have been known to shake our booties at each other : ") Gorillas stick out their tongues to show anger. What does that remind you of? :"). Elephants show affection by entwining their trunks. We all love to cuddle! See, we're not different.

There are many ways to communicate with the animals. Find the one that works for you and practice. The rewards are endless.

Tips on Nutrition and the Health of Our Pets

As part of our family, pets add so much to our lives. Whether it's a friendly face to greet us, a tender brush against a leg, or a gentle nudge, we are constantly reminded of the unconditional love and affection they exude.

Since we have chosen to take them into our homes and our hearts, they look to us for their health and well being. Every pattern in the Universe can also be found replicated in nature. If your pets are restless, ill, unruly, or just plain unhappy; look to yourself first. How does your household run? How can you improve the emotional environment for the entire family, including the critters?

Next, look to the physical environment. Animals are very sensitive to toxins—emotional and physical. Minimize exposure to cleaning products, pesticides, over the counter flea and tick control products, chemical pharmaceuticals, and vaccines. According to Dr. Brandon Brooks, doctor of veterinary medicine and former staff veterinarian of Ask the Vet news forum, "Many (if not most) over the counter (OTC) or non-prescription flea control products are very toxic to cats and kittens- especially the ones only approved for use in dogs. Many people mistakenly buy these for their pet, so it pays to be extra careful when making such a purchase."

According to Dr. Brooks, even though the cat or kitten does not have the OTC flea control product directly applied to it, the cat may still become ill through indirect exposure if it is applied to a dog in the household, household furnishings, bedding, etc. Also, many OTC dog flea control products are toxic to dogs, as well as cats. He does however, offer a healthy alternative. And that is vinegar.

"Vinegar is a naturally occurring germ killer and is one of the very first medicines known to man. It was used as a healing dressing on wounds and infectious sores in Biblical times, and it is credited with saving the lives of thousands of soldiers during the Civil War. It was used routinely as a disinfectant on wounds. It kills germs on contact and it contains bacteria which is unfriendly to infectious microorganisms. It is a natural remedy and most of all, it is safe. Vinegar is particularly useful for neutralizing alkali burns. And it relieves itchy skin too. Coat the 'hot spots' with vinegar, full strength, using a cotton ball or poured directly from the bottle. For a full body treatment, add four cups of vinegar to the bath water. Be careful not to get the vinegar/water mixture in the ears and eyes. The vinegar/water rinses are a quick remedy to relieve minor skin irritations such as hives, chigger bites, other insect bites and rashes."

If you are familiar with my work, you know I am always talking about boosting one immune system or another. This is no different. Our pets need their immune systems kept strong as well. To quote Dr. Rob Robertson, M.D, "Nearly everything that goes wrong with us and our pets, with the exception of trauma - i.e. broken bones, etc., can be traced directly to an immune system failure."

Pollution, drug overload, and nutrient-poor diets compromise our immune health. The key to self-healing is a strong defense system, which protects dogs and cats from everything from the flu germs to cancer cells. Drugs aren't the answer for immune enhancement. The immune system is not responsive to drugs for healing. Antibiotics fight infection, but they don't affect whatever weakened the immune system in the first place.

So, how do we strengthen the immune system? While supplements can be used to support the immune system during any illness, it is most important to keep your pet's immune system acting as healthy as possible all year long

Here are a few suggestions:

1. Feed the most natural diet possible. Learn to read a pet food label and avoid foods with chemical preservatives.
2. Minimize vaccines. Most pets do not need annual "shots." A simple blood test called a titer test can determine which vaccines your pet needs.
3. Eliminate chemicals.
4. Use supplements as needed.
5. Do not use clumping kitty litter. It sticks to their paws, they lick

it off, and it expands inside to cause blockages. Use pine kitty litter that can be dumped in the garden after use and the cats love it. Just like the great outdoors! Clean the litter boxes of solid matter on a daily basis. We flush every time we go. Our feline friends would appreciate the same courtesy.

And most importantly, give them lots of love, kindness and understanding. For sharing their sacred space is an honor we must not take for granted. Honoring each living things' sacred space lives between the in breath and the out breath. We cannot always see its outer boundaries, but the center of its home is nestled in the space between two heartbeats.

How to Discover Your Power Animal Totem or Spirit Guide

Atotem is any natural object, animal or being to whose phenomena and energy you feel closely associated with during your life. The study of animal totems is essential for understanding how the Spiritual world manifests itself within your life, here in the physical. We use these images and energies to learn more about ourselves and our personal contribution to the Universe as a whole. After working with your animals, you will be able to call on their medicines as needed in your own life.

Many ask me how I read so well over the radio waves. The answer to this question is dolphin medicine. I swam with the dolphins, got to know them, and now call on their powers of communication, healing, and fun. The sonar they are so well known for comes in very handy to help me pinpoint where healing is needed. By learning more about the dolphin, I have discovered more about my own gift and how to use it properly. You too, can realize more about yourself and how The Great Mystery works by identifying your power animal totem.

Which animal has always fascinated you? Animals that attract us usually have a lesson for us. What animals do you see most often in your daily life? Do you dream about a certain animal? What animal most frightens you? That which we fear the most is usually what we most need to learn. When we are able to learn that lesson, it becomes a power to us. Have you ever been bitten or attacked by an animal? Shamans believe you gain the medicine of that animal after such an encounter.

Stung by a bee? Maybe you need to get busy. :) I was stung by a jellyfish one summer and now I have the medicine of understanding the value of floating (rather than swimming) through trying emotional times.

Pay attention to the signs from the Universe. All you have to do is be open to the idea and then let it happen. If you would like to know a particular medicine or power a certain animal has for you, check out the Critters page on my web site, www.sandiathey.net. There is a link that will take you to a directory of animals and their messages.

Journal Exercises

I am strongly connected to:

I learn _____ from the animals:

"We shall never know all the good that a simple smile can do."

Mother Teresa

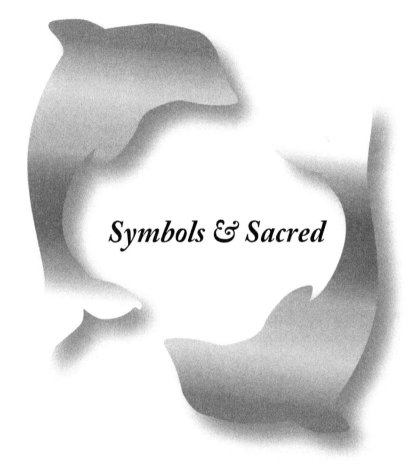

Symbols & Sacred

Finding the Sacred in Everyday Life

J ust as the animals have lessons to teach us, there are many messages in the many aspects of our daily life. In this chapter, we shall explore how symbols can show us the sacred.

How does Earth Mother communicate to us? Through the geometric formations in nature and also through color.

Color can influence our emotions, our actions and how we respond to various people, things and ideas.

Color could be characterized as food for our emotions. Color can increase a sense of well-being, lift the spirits, create a serene setting in which to explore oneself or clarify solutions to everyday problems.

Red symbolizes: action, confidence, courage, vitality
Put some red in your life when you want:
increased enthusiasm and interest, more energy,
action and confidence to go after your dreams,
protection from fears and anxieties.

Pink symbolizes: love, beauty
Put some pink in your life when you want:
calm feelings, to neutralize disorder, bring
relaxation, acceptance, contentment.

Brown symbolizes: earth, order, convention
Put some brown in your life when you want:
a solid wholesome feeling, to blend with the background,
a connection with natural earth and the stability this brings,
orderliness and convention.

Orange symbolizes: vitality with endurance.

Gold symbolizes: wealth, prosperity, wisdom
Put some gold in your life when you want:
increased personal power, relaxation,

enjoyment of life, good health and success.

Yellow symbolizes: wisdom, joy, happiness, intellectual energy
Put some yellow in your life when you want:
clarity for decision-making, relief from 'burnout',
panic, nervousness, exhaustion, sharper memory,
concentration skills, protection from lethargy
and depression during dull weather.

Green symbolizes: life, nature, fertility, well being
Put some green in your life when you want:
a new state of balance, feel a need for change or growth,
freedom to pursue new ideas, protection from fears and anxieties,
connected with the demands of others.

Blue symbolizes: youth, spirituality, truth, peace
Put some blue in your life when you want:
calm and relaxation to counteract chaos or agitation,
to open the flow of communication, to broaden your
perspective in learning new information, solitude and peace

Purple symbolizes: Royalty, magic, mystery
Put some violet in your life when you want:
to use your imagination to its fullest, to re-balance your life,
to remove obstacles, to calm overactivity or to energize
from depression.

White symbolizes: Purity, Cleanliness
Put some white in your life when you want:
to clear clutter and obstacles away, to start a fresh beginning
to bring about mental clarity, purification of thoughts or actions.

Use color in your space, clothes, food, car or computer. Change the color and see what miraculous results you will achieve!

Get inspiration from the greatest artists of all ...The Creator and Earth Mother. Have fun coloring your world!

The Parrot

The parrot is an alert bird with a good temperament. They are very intelligent and have been taught to mimic humans. A bird which can speak the human language is considered to be a link between mankind's world and the world of nature. They're seen as a bridge in which both can cross to gain a deeper understanding about one another. This understanding allows both kingdoms to live in harmony.

One of the most outstanding features of the parrot is its range of coloring. Parrots invoke a sense of hope and promise. Just looking at its brilliant feathers gives us a feeling of excitement and wonder. For those who identify with this totem opportunities to renew their dreams and visions are offered.

Parrots teach us the power of magic. Their feathers are used in healing rituals to invoke the properties of color and light. Color and light therapy have been used by many native tribes to heal the sick or injured. For those with this totem the study of its colors will reveal a lot about yourself.

Parrots can be very vocal or very quiet depending upon the situation they are in. In humans this indicates an innate ability to know when to voice one's opinion and when to be silent. Lessons associated with discernment are always present in a parrot medicine person. The parrot is a feel good bird and is a great ally in healing depression. When the parrot flies into your life, as it has in this chapter, it is asking you to recapture the magic of living. It is time to enjoy your life and all it holds.

The Holidays: Thanksgiving

Throughout history mankind has celebrated the bountiful harvest with thanksgiving ceremonies. Before the establishment of formal religions, many ancient farmers believed that their crops contained spirits which caused the crops to grow and die. Many believed that these spirits would be released when the crops were harvested and they had to be destroyed or they would take revenge on the farmers who harvested them. Some of the harvest festivals celebrated the defeat of these spirits.

Harvest festivals and thanksgiving celebrations were held by the ancient Greeks, the Romans, the Hebrews, the Chinese, and the Egyptians. The ancient Greeks worshipped their goddess of corn, Demeter, who was honored at the festival held each autumn. On the first day of the festival, married women would build leafy shelters and furnish them with couches made with plants. On the second day they fasted. On the third day a feast was held and offerings to the goddess Demeter were made - gifts of seed, corn, cakes, fruit, and pigs. It was hoped that Demeter's gratitude would grant them a good harvest.

The Romans also celebrated a harvest festival called Cerelia, which honored Ceres their goddess of corn (from which the word cereal comes). Their celebration included music, parades, games and sports and a thanksgiving feast. The ancient Egyptians celebrated their harvest festival in honor of Min, their god of vegetation and fertility. The festival was held in the springtime, the Egyptians' harvest season. When the Egyptian farmers harvested their corn, they wept and pretended to be grief-stricken. This was to deceive the spirit which they believed lived in the corn. They feared the spirit would become angry when the farmers cut down the corn where it lived.

In 1621 in the United States, after a hard and devastating first year in the New World, the Pilgrims' fall harvest was very successful and plentiful. Thanks to their Native American teachers, the Pilgrims had beaten the odds. They built homes in the wilderness. They raised enough crops to keep them alive during the long coming winter. Their Governor, William Bradford, proclaimed a day of thanksgiving that was to be shared by all the colonists and the neighboring Native Americans.

In 1817, New York State adopted Thanksgiving Day as an annual custom. Showing gratitude on that special day is important. However, being thankful is something all of us would be well served to adapt as part of our basic nature and express it through our everyday lives. Celebrating the accomplishments of our loved ones, encouraging the potential in ourselves, and living well with joy in our actions are all expressions of thankfulness. The health, happiness and balance of our friends, family, community and world depend on each and every person's contribution to the whole. Remember that the Creator reminds us that blessings are counted in the way that we choose to look at them. Choose wisely.

The Winter Solstice

This is the longest night of the year and the time that we and Earth Mother go into a resting mode. In the pagan religions, on the longest night of the year, the Goddess gives birth to the Sun God and hope for new light is reborn. Yule, as they call it, is a time of awakening to new goals and leaving old regrets behind. Just like our New Year's resolutions! The Christian tradition of a Christmas tree has its origins in the Pagan Yule celebration. Pagan families would bring a live tree into the home so the wood spirits would have a place to keep warm during the cold winter months. Bells were hung in the limbs so you could tell when a spirit was present. The colors of the season, red and green, also are of Pagan origin, as is the custom of exchanging gifts.

And, feeling more emotional these days? Winters are like that: a more inward and sensitive time. According to the Chinese five element system, winter is related to the element of water. And water is what governs our emotions. It's most important to take special care of your kidneys and bladder during the winter. These are the organs most significantly associated with water. They also suggest that blue is an important color for the winter and its link to the water element. You know, deep blue sea, feeling blue? Notice how you are attracted or not to the color. It can direct you to health and balance with your water intake and disposal.

Winter is also a time for preparation while awaiting the greening and rebirth of spring. So, don't worry about those few extra pounds you'll put on this season. There's a reason for it. However, be smart and eat what Mother Nature provides for us. Since Nature's plants are in their deepest parts, take advantage and eat rooted vegetables like carrots, turnips, onions and potatoes. And nuts are a great winter snack! Spices like cayenne pepper and ginger are also warming on those cold nights. Arbonne knows this and has an amazing ginger citrus line they introduce in the winter: including teas, scrubs and lotions.

Remember, we are a part of this cycle. Not observers. The more you go with the flow and with what God has provided for us through the Earth, the happier and healthier you are. Flow through this winter. Find a cozy spot to relax, sleep and dream. A little more rest is beneficial during this time. Let's all enjoy a little bear medicine. They sure do know how to hibernate!

Winter is an important time to feel what your inner changes are and weave them into your dance of existence.

Origins of Halloween

Halloween is an annual celebration, but just what is it actually a celebration of? And how did this peculiar custom originate? Is it, as some claim, a kind of demon worship? Or is it just a harmless vestige of some ancient pagan ritual?

This information comes from a paper by Dr. Jerry Wilson. The word itself, "Halloween," actually has its origins in the Catholic Church. It comes from a contracted corruption of All Hallows Eve. November 1, "All Hollows Day" (or All Saints Day), is a Catholic day of observance in honor of saints. In the 5th century BC, in Celtic Ireland, summer officially ended on October 31. The holiday was called Samhain (sow-en), the Celtic New Year."

One story says that, on that day, the disembodied spirits of all those who had died throughout the preceding year, would come back in search of living bodies to possess for the next year. It was believed to be their only hope for the afterlife. The Celts believed all laws of space and time were suspended during this time, allowing the spirit world to intermingle with the living. Naturally, the living did not want to be possessed. So on the night of October 31, villagers would extinguish the fires in their homes, to make them cold and undesirable. They would then dress up in all manner of ghoulish costumes and noisily paraded around the neighborhood. They thought being as destructive as possible would frighten away spirits looking for bodies to possess.

The thrust of the practices also changed over time to become more ritualized. As belief in spirit possession waned, the practice of dressing up like hobgoblins, ghosts, and witches took on a more ceremonial role. The custom of Halloween was brought to America in the 1840s by Irish immigrants fleeing their country's potato famine. At that time, the favorite pranks in New England included tipping over outhouses and unhinging fence gates.

The custom of trick-or-treating is thought to have originated not with the Irish Celts, but with a ninth-century European custom called souling. On November 2, All Souls Day, early Christians would walk from village to village begging for "soul cakes," made out of square pieces of

bread with currants. The more soul cakes the beggars would receive, the more prayers they would promise to say on behalf of the dead relatives of the donors. At the time, it was believed that the dead remained in limbo for a time after
death and that prayer, even by strangers, could expedite a soul's passage to heaven.

The Jack-o-lantern custom probably comes from Irish folklore. As the tale is told, a man named Jack, who was notorious as a drunkard and trickster, tricked Satan into climbing a tree. Jack then carved an image of a cross in the tree's trunk, trapping the devil up the tree. Jack made a deal with the devil: if he would never tempt him again, he would promise to let him down the tree. According to the folk tale, after Jack died, he was denied entrance to Heaven because of his evil ways. He was also denied access to Hell because he had tricked the devil. Instead, the devil gave him a single ember to light his way through the frigid darkness. The ember was placed inside a hollowed-out turnip to keep it glowing longer. When the immigrants came to America, they found that pumpkins were far more plentiful than turnips.

The day itself did not grow out of evil practices. It grew out of the rituals of Celts celebrating a new year and out of medieval, prayer rituals of Europeans. And, of course, whatever you believe, make the most of it and connect to the joyous energy of the day. Even if you are just celebrating being alive!!!!

"Time and money spent in helping men to do more for themselves is far better than mere giving."
Henry Ford

Hanukkah

Hanukkah, the festival of lights. Hanukkah has a profound spiritual significance - celebrating the reemergence of light in a time of darkness, of freedom in a time of tyranny, of hope and rededication in a time of despair. And we learn something about conservation of the earth's resources — especially of oil — from the story of how the Temple's rededication was achieved when one bottle of sacred oil — one day's worth — lasted for eight days until more oil could be obtained. This is why we celebrate eight days of Hanukkah. This conservation of oil was a Divine miracle.

We might translate this to mean that it is a sacred act, carrying out God's will and following God's lead, for us to conserve oil, trees, water, air — all the strands of earth. To conserve, to renew, to heal. In order to do this we must all have a common vision: starting with reaching out to help another. Whether that be a two-legged, an animal or the Earth. By sharing our gifts and having gratitude for what we have...anything is possible.

Let's all celebrate the festival of lights by bringing out the light in ourselves and passing that on to others. Reach out, be of service and the Creator will make you last a lifetime.

Memorial Day

Memorial Day, originally called Decoration Day, is a day of remembrance for those who have died in our nation's service. Memorial Day was officially proclaimed on May 5, 1868 by General John Logan, national commander of the Grand Army of the Republic. It was first observed on May 30, 1868, when flowers were placed on the graves of Union and Confederate soldiers at Arlington National Cemetery.

The first state to officially recognize the holiday was New York in 1873. By 1890 it was recognized by all of the northern states. The South refused to acknowledge the day, honoring their dead on separate days until after World War I (when the holiday changed from honoring just those who died fighting in the Civil War to honoring Americans who died fighting in any war). It is now celebrated in almost every state on the last Monday in May.

So what happens on a spiritual level when all these people are thinking about death? When two or more are gathered in my name, strength in numbers, the more the merrier...there is power in collective energy. We all know this. On Memorial Day, when great numbers of people are remembering and honoring the dead, it opens a space for those spirits and that death energy to be activated. It can affect each one of us differently. We may have a melancholy feeling about a recent loss. The ghosts of those souls who haven't passed properly may visit us. We may have strange dreams or déjà vu.

So what do we do about it to make a positive impact? Tap into the energy of love and acceptance to help them pass. Before you have your picnic, take a moment to be silent and add to the intention of honoring all of those who have died in service. Wish them safe journeys and appreciate their contribution to the whole. Then honor all who have passed, and honor the Universe, by being joyful and grateful for being alive.

Autumn

As the days shorten, the nights grow longer and everyone prepares for the holidays, it occurred to me that it's important for us to understand the impact this glorious season. The leaves are changing and the air feels a bit crisper. The fall equinox is the first day of autumn and signifies balance. On this date both day and night are equal. 12 hours of each.

The astrological sign Libra also begins the autumnal equinox. Libra's symbol is a scale, representing the balance of light and dark. Mythically, this is the day of the year when the God of light is defeated by his twin and alter-ego - the God of Darkness. There are many common themes throughout the fall holidays. It's all about abundance, balance, harvesting, and remembrance.

Ancient Celts conducted a mock sacrifice of a wicker-work figure which represented the vegetation Spirit as an offer of thanksgiving to their God. The Christian Church replaced the fall Pagan solstice celebrations during medieval time with Michaelmas, the feast of the Archangel Michael. The Mayans constructed a pyramid which displayed patterns of light at the time of the solstice. The dates signaled the start of a harvest planting, or a religious ceremony.

March 17th – Wearin' of the Green

May God grant you always...A sunbeam to warm you, a moonbeam to charm you, a sheltering Angel so nothing can harm you. Laughter to cheer you. Faithful friends near you. And whenever you pray, Heaven to hear you.

Happy St. Patrick's Day

The Daily Dance

"April showers bring May flowers"
Thomas Tusser

Put a Little Spring in Your Step: April

April was the second month in an early Roman calendar, but became the fourth when the ancient Romans started using January as the first month. The Romans called the month Aprilis. It may come from a word meaning 'to open', or it may come from Aphrodite, the Greek name for the goddess of love.

Some facts about April

Samuel Morey patented the internal combustion engine
on April 1, 1826.

Apple Computer was formed by Steve Jobs and Steve Wozniak
on April 1, 1976.

The United States Mint was established on April 2, 1792.

Martin Luther King Jr. delivered his
"I've Been to the Mountaintop" speech on April 3, 1968.

The Beatles occupied the top five positions on the Billboard
Hot 100 pop chart on April 4, 1964.

Warner Bros. premiered the first 3-D film, House of Wax,
on April 9, 1953.

Yuri Gagarin became the first human to travel into
outer space on April 12, 1961.

Videotape was first demonstrated on April 14, 1956.

The first crossword puzzle book was published on April 18, 1924.

The Daily Dance

April cold with dropping rain
Willows and lilacs brings again,
The whistle of returning birds
And trumpet-lowing of the herds.
Ralph Waldo Emerson

'Spring is nature's way of saying, 'Let's party!' "
Robin Williams

Unknown Speaker addressing the National Congress of American Indians in the mid 1960s:

"In early days we were close to nature. We judged time, weather conditions, and many things by the elements – the good earth, the blue sky, the flying of geese, and the changing winds. We looked to these for guidance and answers. Our prayers and thanksgiving were said to the four winds – to the East, from whence the new day was born; to the South, which sent the warm breeze which gave a feeling of comfort; to the West, which ended the day and brought rest; and to the North, the Mother of winter whose sharp air awakened a time of preparation for the long days ahead. We lived by God's hand through nature and evaluated the changing winds to tell us or warn us of what was ahead.

Today, we are again evaluating the changing winds. May we be strong in spirit and equal to our Fathers of another day in reading the signs accurately and interpreting them wisely. May Wah-Kon-Tah, the Great Spirit, look down upon us, guide us, inspire us, and give us courage and wisdom. Above all, may He look down upon us and be pleased."

Echo says Hello!!!

There are many beliefs about the dolphins. To the early Christians, the dolphin was a symbol of salvation. To the Greeks, it was a sacred messenger of the gods. Echo, a dolphin is my personal animal totem.

Dolphins have a purity of being which touches our inner nature. We want to swim with them, observe them, have them entertain us, play with them, and, yes, because of their keen minds and helpful nature, we look to them for healing.

There was even an entire television series starring a dolphin! Kindness, play, savior, guide, sea power, intelligence, communication, and charity. They live their life in joyful harmony with each other and their world. They seem to have learned the lesson that love is the most important part of life.

Our communication to you today via the dolphins is:

ee..eee...ee..eee from the Daily Dance

In Closing

May our tips have reached you in the way you needed.

May our segments have put joy in your heart and a smile on your face.

May all of our intentions have respectively penetrated your space with healing and growth.

Acknowledgements

The acknowledgements for this book are as vast and infinite as the Universe itself. First and foremost my appreciation for The Creator, Earth Mother, Grandmother Moon, Grandfather Sun, all the Directions, The Animals, my spirit guides, all the souls in every dimension that have supported and encouraged me…my heartfelt gratitude is wealthy and abundant.

The kindness and attention of the many energies during my journey here on Earth are extra special and I thank them all for their love and companionship. Each in their own way has contributed to the teachings and lessons in the daily dance of my life.

Thank you to:

Michael Pincus for showing the love, sharing the love and being the love.

My brother, Andrew for being there with his wise and caring nature. And for sharing his beautiful family, Erinn, Sasha, Keegan, Hunter and Samantha with me.

Melinda Paul for all the sister adventures.

My best friend and companion, Gray Kitty for her patience and loyalty.

Huge hugs of grateful joy to Kathy Connolly and her parents, Ann and Tommy. Also to Dr. Dan Nattell, Jerry Stringham and all my friends from Delmar.

Expansive thoughts of appreciation to Carol Stover, Pam Miller, Tara Hannon, Ken Rochon, Vince Sharps, Glenn Klausner, Thunderbear, Karen Blackburn, Ron Markwood, Mike Ruby, Linda Soares, Steve Baron, Emily LaLumia, Linda Lowry, Allen Troutman and the Treehouse, Jerry McLean,

Daily Dance

Dr. Wanda Ramsey, Hot Guest, WCBM,
Charlie & Ernie & Lisa, WVMT, my esteemed co-host, Tony Pann,
Shari Hammond, Kate Rubino and my Jewish Mother,
Miriam Bernstein.

The love and appreciation I have for Jeffrey Applebaum, The Rock Man is in a category all his own with the Black Hills and the buffalo.

Thank you to Maureen O'Crean for the connection, guidance and hours of attention that went into creating *The Daily Dance*.

I am also extremely appreciative that Heather Nelson put her special touch of love on this book.

My life has been blessed with special people doing extraordinary things and for that I am truly grateful. Thank you.

133

About Sandi Athey

For most of us, human beings that is, we come to a place in the road where we ask, *How did I end up here?* Without judgment, our journey is our journey with all the twists and turns of a good movie or a novel. Some of our destinations are created by our brilliant thinking, others by our mistakes. Some of our stops are joyful, others are fraught with pain. No one escapes this trip on life's train without a story. My story and journey, though most likely different from yours, took a detour that led me here, on the page with you, and I'll get back to that one in a moment.

If you looked at the images of my life, you would see a young, ambitious woman in her 30's working to make her mark in the world. I was a top selling insurance agent with money to burn, drove a hot car and paid no attention to my physical body other than getting to the gym. I burned the candle at both ends and on one fateful night in Olney, Maryland, my life's train came to an abrupt halt when I was killed by an attacker, known at that time as the Route 29 Corridor serial rapist. The moment when I left my body is seared into my memory, as well as seeing my attacker from the other side. It was eerie and peaceful all at the same time, exactly like watching a movie, a horror movie, but a movie none-the-less.

Like most evenings, I was working late and felt quite safe and secure in my office. It was in a good part of town, but something always nagged at me to make sure that my office mate always locked the door at 5:00. Today I would say that was my intuition trying to break through, but I didn't believe in things like that back then. I do now.

He opened the unlocked front door and made his way to my office. I was getting ready to leave for the night and when I opened my door, there he was. In a split second he had me and as he was choking me, I knew I was dead when the pain stopped. I could see him from the other side, he was shocked that his brutal actions had killed me, a new escalation of his crimes. Up until this night he had raped and beatened numerous other women, who lived through the ordeal and he had always successfully evaded the police.

While I was watching his actions from the other side, I saw his back and white sneakers when he kicked me. God as I know him said, "You know you have to go back, you have work to do." To tell you the truth I did not want to go back. Wherever I was, some people think it is heaven, all I knew is that I wanted to stay in the light. I also knew that a world of hurt awaited that broken body that was me, lying on the floor. But go back I did and my chest exploded as my body fought to breathe again and I began dragging myself across the floor to call 911 with my last bit of strength. The police came and I lived to get a new start and a new destination on my life's train.

Eventually he was caught and put on trial. I shared my story with the authorities and was instructed not to talk about being on the other side. During the trial, the prosecuting attorney held up a paper bag and asked me to describe what footwear my attacker was wearing. As I described the sneakers I saw from the other side, she pulled them out of the bag and the entire courtroom gasped. It felt good to have my experience validated. The only thing left to do was lock the cell door behind him for a very, very long time.

So why do I tell you my story? So that you will know you are not alone. That bad things happen to good people and the only thing you can do is get on with the life that you are destined to live; one of gratitude, beauty, joy, love and hope. As I could put the attack behind me, I went through a process of healing; my body, mind, emotions and spirit. I began to eat organic food and discover healthful ways of living. I embraced a course of study in the ways of the Native Americans and started to accept the gift I had been given on that fateful night, of being psychic. I am able to see the many realms of our lives and to discover the blocks that keep us from moving forward. I am often visited by those who have passed before us and for 7 years on The Psychic Healing radio show I answered questions from where have I put my glasses? to do I have a medical issue and need to see my doctor? I learned that using my gifts to tell the future was not a path for me, because your future is soundly in your hands, so make good decisions. I took hold of my intuition and embraced that there are many mysteries in this marvelous Universe we share with Mother Earth and The Creator and we are here to learn, with joy.

It is always an honor for me to share my life lessons and your life lessons with you in our private sessions, on the radio and through this book, The Daily Dance. And with the words of that most ancient prophet, Star Trek's Mr. Spock, "Live Long and Prosper."*

I wish you joy, blessings for a life fulfilled and most of all, live happily ever after.

Safe journeys and I'll talk to you soon,
Sandi Athey
Spirit of the Wind Director
Institute of Happily Ever After

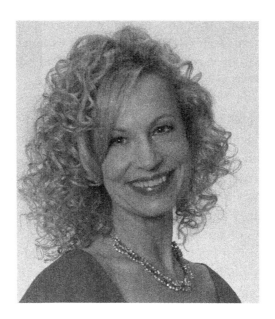

Sandi Athey

References

Thank you to these wonderful resources

www.albany.edu/~dp1252/isp523/halloween.html
Amazon facts, psychicsandi.amazonherb.net
Animal Speak by Ted Andrews
www.askavetquestion.com
The Bible
www.drstandley.com
Earth Medicine by Jamie Sams
www.edgarcayce.org
www.explore-old-west-colorado.com/native-scarred-trees.html
www.firstpeople.us/FP-Html-Legends/TwoWolves-Cherokee.html
www.history.com
kims3003.hubpages.com/hub/Colors-What-They-Mean-What-
www.myjewishlearning.com/holidays/Jewish_Holidays/Hanukkah/History.
shtml
Star Wars by George Lucas
talking-feather.com/2009/12/24/walking-in-beauty-a-navajo-prayer/
Time Magazine August 4, 2003
The Wizard of Oz by L. Frank Baum
thethoughtsoftracy.blogspot.com/2009/08/split-apart-theory.html
www.themystica.com/mystica/articles/e/esp_extrasensory_perception.html
ww.usmemorialday.org/backgrnd.html
www.wikipedia.org

To contact Sandi:

Please visit www.sandiathey.net

By Mail:

Sandi Athey c/o
Distinctively Diva Press
703 Pier Avenue, Ste B. #309
Hermosa Beach, CA 90254
By Phone:

410-747-6510

By Email:

psychicsandi@cs.com

Sandi is available to speak to your group and organization. Please contact her at the above addresses for more information

CPSIA information can be obtained
at www.ICGtesting.com
Printed in the USA
BVOW06s0317220317

479130BV00006B/13/P